PRAISE FOR *HEART ATTACK PROOF*

"Dr. Michael Ozner has written another splendid book! If all of us heeded to his recommendations, atherosclerotic plaques (blockages, hardening of the arteries) would be prevented or shrink, and heart attacks and brain attacks would occur far less commonly. We have the power to prevent the most common cause of death in the Western world, and Dr. Ozner shows us step-by-step just how to do it. Thank you, Dr. O!"

—WILLIAM C. ROBERTS, MD, *Editor in Chief, The American Journal of Cardiology, and Medical Director, Baylor Heart and Vascular Institute, Baylor University Medical Center*

———

"Read and become *Heart Attack Proof*—the essential guide to achieving immunity from America's number one killer. And, after you finish the book, pass it on to save even more lives!"

—PHILIP SMITH, *Editor in Chief,* Life Extension Magazine

———

"In his book, *Heart Attack Proof*, Dr. Michael Ozner takes the reader on a six-week journey that leads to a 'cardiac makeover' and a lifetime of optimal heart-health. What distinguishes *Heart Attack Proof* from similar works in this field is Dr. Ozner's ability to translate sound principles of preventive cardiology into simple, practical, sustainable changes that lead readers to a 'new normal' way of living. Rather than a program built on rigid dietary restrictions and aggressive 'no pain, no gain' exercise recommendations, this book meets individuals where they are and provides step-wise options to facilitate successful change. It is my pleasure to recommend *Heart Attack Proof* for anyone looking for a real world approach to achieving a sustainable heart healthy lifestyle."

—WILLIAM CROMWELL, MD, FAHA, FNLA, *Chief, Lipoprotein and Metabolic Disorders Institute, Wake Forest University School of Medicine*

———

"Dr. Ozner's new book, *Heart Attack Proof*, is a must-read for all health-conscious individuals interested in information to help reduce the risk of heart disease or stroke. Dr. Ozner represents the best in modern medicine, a compassionate and highly respected cardiologist, intimately familiar with subtle and complex medical science, yet able to distill down and communicate critical information in an understandable way to his patients. If you want to know how to *prevent* a heart attack, read this book—now!"

—STEVEN V. JOYAL, MD, *Chief Medical Officer, Life Extension, Inc.*

Michael Ozner, MD

Heart Attack Proof

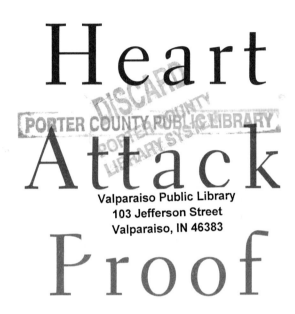

A Six-Week Cardiac Makeover for a Lifetime of Optimal Health

BenBella

Copyright © 2012 by Michael Ozner, MD
Color lab reports used with permission from HDL, Inc.

BenBella Books, Inc.
10300 N. Central Expressway, Suite 400
Dallas, TX 75231
www.benbellabooks.com
Send feedback to feedback@benbellabooks.com

Printed in the United States of America
10 9 8 7 6 5 4 3 2 1
Library of Congress Cataloging-in-Publication Data is available for this title.
978-1-936661-85-5

Copyediting by Oriana Leckert
Proofreading by Michael Fedison
Cover design by Faceout Studio
Text design and composition by John Reinhardt Book Design
Printed by Bang Printing

Distributed by Perseus Distribution
(www.perseusdistribution.com)
To place orders through Perseus Distribution:
Tel: 800-343-4499
Fax: 800-351-5073
E-mail: orderentry@perseusbooks.com

Significant discounts for bulk sales are available.
Please contact Glenn Yeffeth at glenn@benbellabooks.com or (214) 750-3628.

To my wife Christine and my children Jennifer and Jonathan:

You are my heart and soul.

Contents

Foreword...ix

Acknowledgments...xi

Introduction...1

WEEK 1: Begin Your Cardiac Makeover.....................5

WEEK 2: Get Fit for Life......................................19

WEEK 3: Create a Stress-Free Lifestyle...................35

WEEK 4: Achieve Optimal Nutrition.......................55

WEEK 5: Know Your Numbers...............................89

WEEK 6: Heart-Healthy Supplements....................141

             Heart Attack Proof—At Last!...................153

             Appendices..155

APPENDIX A: Body Mass Index (BMI) Chart............156

APPENDIX B: Omega-3 (EPA and DHA) Content in Fish
and Fish Oil......................................157

APPENDIX C: A Heart-Healthy 7-Day Meal Plan.......160

APPENDIX D: The Restaurant Survival Guide...........198

APPENDIX E: National Cholesterol Guidelines..........200

APPENDIX F: Advanced Cardiovascular Diagnostic Tests........207

Bibliography and Additional Reading.................252

About the Author..268

Index...269

Foreword

HEART DISEASE is the number-one killer in the world, and in the United States cardiovascular disease deaths nearly outnumber deaths from all other causes combined. This, however, does not have to be the case. Evidence now demonstrates that atherosclerosis—the process that leads to heart attack and stroke—can be halted and even reversed, suggesting that heart disease can be beaten!

The notion that we can beat heart disease is supported by the fact that in recent years significant progress has been made in diagnosis and treatment, resulting in a decline in the percentage of cardiovascular events (heart attacks, strokes, etc.) per capita. This success can be attributed to the development of new drugs, like statins, which lower low-density lipoprotein (LDL), and new antihypertensive agents, which decrease blood pressure, in addition to educational programs promoting smoking cessation and a healthy lifestyle. Unfortunately, this progress has been counteracted by even more insidious disorders: diabetes and the metabolic syndrome, the prevalence of which has been significantly increasing over the past several years. Since individuals with diabetes have an equivalent risk of future cardiovascular events as individuals diagnosed with heart disease, our net progress in the fight against heart disease may actually be nil, or even negative.

With all of our increasing knowledge, why are we continuing to lose the battle against heart disease? To better understand this, it is important to realize that heart disease does not have a single cause. Rather, it is a multifactorial disorder with many contributing factors stemming from environmental, biochemical, socioeconomic, stress-related, and genetic causes. Therefore, we cannot simply focus just on our cholesterol levels, but need to consider other quantifiable contributors influenced both by genetics and by individual behavior. The Mayo Brothers, who founded the Mayo Clinic where I had the distinguished pleasure to train and practice for fourteen years, were truly visionaries in this regard. They developed the idea of group practice, in which several physicians with expertise in different areas work as a team to identify and appropriately address multiple, often interrelated disease processes occurring in each individual patient. This visionary approach changed the field of medical practice in the United States and propelled the Mayo Clinic, which started as a small practice in rural Minnesota, to become the most renowned medical institution in the world.

Dr. Michael Ozner continues to further the advancement of this same idea in this book, by addressing the numerous contributing causes of heart disease. What separates Dr. Ozner's approach from the other heart disease prevention books on the market is that, rather than focusing only on one element—just on diet or just on cholesterol—he shows you how to address the full range of lifestyle and metabolic factors essential to heart disease, using the most up-to-date medical tests available.

In short, Dr. Ozner paves a path that confronts the complexities of heart disease on all fronts and that, if followed, will enable you to reverse heart disease progression. It will take some effort on your part, as well as consultation with your physician and other medical professionals, but if you follow the simple and straightforward guidelines set forth by Dr. Ozner in this book, you can indeed become Heart Attack Proof!

JOSEPH P. MCCONNELL, PhD, DABCC
Director of Cardiovascular Laboratory Medicine
The Mayo Clinic, Rochester, Minnesota: 1998–2009
Chief Medical Officer and Laboratory Director
Health Diagnostic Laboratory, Inc., Richmond, Virginia: 2009–present

Acknowledgments

I would like to thank my patients and colleagues who gave me the inspiration and motivation to write *Heart Attack Proof*. I am especially grateful to the following individuals, who have taken extensive time and effort to review and critique *Heart Attack Proof*: Joseph P. McConnell, PhD, Laboratory Director, Health Diagnostic Laboratory; William C. Roberts, MD, Editor-in-Chief, *The American Journal of Cardiology*, and Medical Director, Baylor Heart and Vascular Institute, Baylor University Medical Center; William Cromwell, MD, FAHA, FNLA, Chief, Lipoprotein and Metabolic Disorders Institute; and Philip Smith, Editor-in-Chief, *Life Extension* magazine. In addition, I would like to thank Aimee Dingwell for her editorial assistance.

I would also like to acknowledge all the nurse educators who share my passion for cardiovascular disease prevention, and who have helped me organize and promote the Wellness & Prevention program at Baptist Health South Florida. This program provides education and prevention strategies for patients who have cardiovascular disease and for those with risk factors for heart disease. I would also like to express my appreciation of Brian Keeley, CEO of Baptist Health South Florida, for allowing me to conduct an annual Cardiovascular Disease Prevention Symposium dedicated to the treatment and prevention of heart attack and stroke. In addition, I am grateful to the wonderful Medical Education Department at Baptist Health South Florida for supporting and assisting me in the organization and planning of this widely attended international symposium.

I am also grateful to Glenn Yeffeth (publisher) and Leah Wilson (editor) at BenBella Books for their steadfast guidance and advice.

Finally, and most importantly, I would like to thank my wife, Christine Ozner, RN, who has a special interest in heart disease prevention through nutrition and exercise, and has contributed immensely to the editing of this book.

Introduction

On June 13, 2008, the NBC newsroom in Washington, D.C., was functioning as it always does. There was hustling and bustling, researchers gathering details on any breaking news, and interns running messages to and fro. Meanwhile, in typical lighthearted fashion, Bureau Chief and *Meet the Press* host Tim Russert was recording voice-overs with colleagues for his Sunday show.

But shortly after 1:30 p.m., in the middle of his work, Russert collapsed. Despite having coronary artery disease that was being managed with medication and exercise—his LDL, or bad cholesterol, was at 68 mg/dl, which is below the recommended threshold of 70 mg/dl—Russert died suddenly from a heart attack.

"How could this be?" you may wonder. It's a question many of us in the medical community asked as well. Since Russert's passing was so well publicized, we learned more details about his cardiovascular profile, most notably that his HDL, or good cholesterol level, was risky at 37 mg/dl, though it was below the recommended metric of 40 mg/dl for a man. In addition, he had a history of hypertension and diabetes.

Russert's death received national attention, but the sad truth is that thousands of needless, premature deaths from heart attack happen every day. Based on current data, the majority of you reading this book—at least those of you who continue to adhere to the typical American diet and lifestyle, full of highly processed foods, low in physical exertion, and high in daily stress—will probably die from a heart attack. That is not fear-mongering; it's a statistical fact. For decades, heart disease has been the number one cause of death in the United States. *But it doesn't have to be so.* Coronary heart disease is preventable, even reversible, which means future heart attacks are also preventable. While heart disease has become the leading killer of our time, it *can* be defeated.

If heart disease is so preventable, why has it become an epidemic? It's partly due to the toxic American diet, which is highly processed, calorie-dense, and nutrient-depleted. We too often choose convenience and elaborate packaging over the traditional food options of days past, like whole fruits and vegetables, nuts and grains, and fish rich in omega-3. What we've learned in the last few years is that these foods not only give us great nutrition, but they have specific ingredients that can protect us from heart disease.

But it's more than the foods we choose to eat that matters. We can't forget the impact of the context in which we eat that food. Consider just one day in the lives of two men similar in age: Ted and Giovanni.

It was a typical day for Ted. He awoke at 6 A.M. and had his usual breakfast of bacon, eggs, and fried potatoes. He left home in a hurry after an argument with his wife and drove to his office to begin another stressful day as a real estate executive. At a 9:30 A.M. board meeting, he presented a proposal for purchasing a large office complex. During the meeting he had coffee and doughnuts and smoked several cigarettes. It was customary for Ted to argue with his partners, and today was no different. After several phone calls he was off to the airport to catch a noon flight. He had no time to sit down for lunch, so he drove to his favorite fast-food drive-through for a burger and fries, which he ate quickly while on the way to the airport. After parking his car and walking briskly to the terminal, he developed crushing chest pain and broke into a sweat. He grabbed a roll of Tums from his pocket and chewed several tablets. The pain subsided, but then returned with a vengeance several minutes later. This time it was an intense pressure in his chest, which radiated to his arms and his jaw. He had a feeling of impending doom as he collapsed at the security gate and lost consciousness. Later, he awoke in a nearby emergency room, having been resuscitated by paramedics. It was clear that Ted had suffered a massive heart attack and was lucky to be alive. Following an extensive hospital stay with heart catheterization and coronary bypass surgery, Ted's life would never be the same.

Giovanni awoke the same day in his small Italian village. He had a light breakfast of whole grain bread with jam and fruit. He walked to his office and had a pleasant morning conversing with clients of his import/export business. At 2:00 P.M. he returned home and had an enjoyable lunch with family and friends. Lunch consisted of a salad with olive oil, whole-wheat pasta, whole grain bread, garlic, goat cheese, red wine, and fresh fruit. Following lunch, he rested for an hour before returning to work.

Was Ted's heart attack preventable? Is Giovanni's good health a matter of luck? The answer seems crystal clear—and the science supports it. A healthy diet along with prudent exercise and regular relaxation are key contributors to a long life of good health.

The approach in this book is the one that I have utilized in my preventive cardiology practice for more than twenty-five years to significantly reduce the risk of heart attack and stroke in my patients. Now I'm making it available to you. Science has progressed a lot over the last quarter century; our understanding of what causes heart disease has evolved, more studies have been done, and new laboratory tests are now letting us uncover previously hidden risk. But the best, most effective approach to preventing heart attack and stroke hasn't changed at all. The latest science has just confirmed it.

If we are smart and committed to change, in the majority of circumstances, we have the tools to prevent coronary heart disease. In the pages that follow, I'll guide you on a six-week journey through the lifestyle and medical changes necessary to achieve optimum heart health. Each week we'll build on the previous week's tasks, until you've achieved a full cardiac makeover. Embracing these prevention principles and developing a heart disease prevention plan with your personal physician will allow you to take control of your health and begin your journey to becoming virtually Heart Attack Proof.

Begin Your Cardiac Makeover

Prevention is better than the cure.

—DESIDERIUS ERASMUS
fifteenth-century philosopher

W HEN I FIRST MET SUZANNE, she was a seemingly healthy patient. A teacher in her late forties with a teenage daughter, she wasn't the face of heart disease. She was of normal weight and clearly living an active and productive life. But inside, something was brewing. She had already suffered a mild heart attack, and had undergone several angioplasties before she came to me seeking help. Her husband had been tragically killed in a car accident several years before, and now, as a single mother and widow, Suzanne was terrified. What if the treatments and medications didn't work and she had another heart attack? What if she didn't survive? "Who will raise my daughter?" she asked me. "What can I do?"

If you have asked yourself the same questions and had no way to answer them, I have great news for you: There is much you can do to maintain good health and prevent cardiovascular disease. I'm going to tell you how.

Chances are that if you're reading this right now, you are frightened of the same sort of what-ifs that Suzanne was. The hard truth is that you likely have good reason to be. Heart disease is the number one killer in the United States, regardless of gender. And heart disease kills more people each year than all cancers combined. The majority of you reading this book will die of cardiovascular disease (whether heart attack or stroke) if you don't change your current lifestyle. The amazing thing is that heart disease isn't the inevitable consequence of aging. We know what to do to prevent it. And we now know how to reverse it!

Unfortunately, our modern "go, go, go" world has become "bad, bad, bad" for our health and wreaked havoc on our bodies. Processed foods designed to be "fast" and "convenient" are loaded with saturated fat, trans fat, salt, and refined sugar, and are devoid of essential nutrients. Yet they've replaced the best foods we can eat—whole, natural foods that are loaded with essential nutrients, healthy fiber, and free radical–fighting antioxidants.

Technological advances, while keeping us connected, have rendered us desk- or couch-bound, sedentary and stressed. We've forgotten how positively uplifting movement and flexibility is. The result? More and more of us are facing obesity, diabetes, heart disease, cancer, and that inevitable question: "What if . . . ?"

Fortunately, we have learned much over the last two decades. Important, life-saving research has shown that you can *prevent and even reverse* heart disease, and live without the fear of succumbing prematurely to a heart attack.

Let's get back to Suzanne. I started her on my prevention plan—the one you'll find in the pages of this book. She changed her diet, started walking regularly, began meditation, and quit smoking. With lifestyle changes and cholesterol-lowering medication, she significantly lowered her bad (LDL) cholesterol and raised her good (HDL) cholesterol. She normalized the number of bad (atherogenic) particles in her blood and decreased the markers of vascular inflammation. Most importantly, she regained hope. She realized that she had control of her destiny—and she became healthier and happier to boot! Twelve years later, when she came to my office for a routine annual follow-up, she was smiling and had tears of joy in her eyes as she showed me pictures of her daughter's wedding.

So get ready. Over the next six weeks I'll lead you through a complete cardiac makeover. Even if you've been told you have hypertension or hypercholesterolemia, or have already undergone stent insertion or bypass surgery, this book is the key to unlocking the door to a healthier life.

Assignment #1: Take a Mediterranean Vacation... From Your Toxic American Diet!

Your first task is to take an inventory of your diet. Hamburgers, hot dogs, macaroni and cheese, ice cream, French fries...are they on your shopping list? What are your favorite foods? Which foods do you always purchase? Take notes when you shop.

Food is the single most important factor influencing your overall health. It's also a factor you have *complete* control over. Moreover, we are learning which foods can truly protect us and which foods can be devastating to our health.

Not all foods are created equal, and many of the foods that make up a traditional Western diet are toxic to our bodies. Consuming unhealthy food is like putting diesel fuel in a gasoline-powered car—it simply does not work. We are not genetically programmed to function on processed food! In fact, processed food is directly related to today's ever-increasing trend toward obesity, hypertension, diabetes, heart disease, stroke, and yes, death.

The toxic American diet is loaded with preservatives, sodium, refined sugar, and bad fats. So what's the alternative? Become

IF I BECOME "HEART ATTACK PROOF," CAN I STILL HAVE A HEART ATTACK?

When you buckle your seat belt, you greatly reduce your risk of serious injury or death resulting from an automobile accident. Likewise, by starting your cardiac makeover and becoming Heart Attack Proof you will significantly lower your risk of a heart attack. Yes, it is still possible to have a heart attack despite following the heart-health information in this book, but the likelihood will be greatly reduced. Using this book as a guide, sit down with your personal physician and discuss a prevention plan that will lead to a lifetime of optimal health and happiness. You control your destiny!

Mediterranean! Begin a healthy, delicious, and nutritious dietary plan complete with colorful fruits and vegetables, whole grain bread and pasta, omega-3-rich seafood, and red wine.

For many years I had been intrigued as to why people living near the Mediterranean Sea are by all accounts healthier than their American counterparts. Despite a less advanced medical system, significantly fewer people were dying from heart attacks, strokes, or cancer, or suffering from chronic conditions like diabetes or Alzheimer's disease. The evidence for why this is points almost exclusively to diet and lifestyle.

Study after study has shown that those following a traditional Mediterranean diet suffer significantly less heart disease and are far less likely to die from a heart attack than those following a traditional American diet. In fact, one of the oldest studies, the Seven Countries Study, showed that Greek men living on the island of Crete were more than 80 percent less likely to die from a heart attack than their American counterparts.

But even more compelling is research showing that those who *switch* to a Mediterranean diet and lifestyle share the same health benefits (including fewer heart attacks and a longer life expectancy), regardless of where they live or what their diets were like before. Why?

We know that there are certain foods and food components that can change your cardiovascular disease risk. There are literally dozens of "super foods" in the Mediterranean diet that are absolute musts to start eating—not only because they are good for you, but because they taste great too!

For now, take note of what you're eating and start stocking up on Mediterranean favorites. We'll talk more about the Mediterranean diet and embark on a heart-healthy 7-day meal plan in Week 4.

As Dr. Ancel Keyes, a noted epidemiologist of the last century and author of the Seven Countries Study, put it, "If some developed countries can do without heart attacks, why can't we?"

A FEW MEDITERRANEAN MUSTS

Try these heart-healthy foods instead of their toxic alternatives:

Try	Instead of
Oatmeal	Sugary cereal
Almonds	Potato chips
Grilled salmon	Grilled steak
Fresh fruit	Cheese cake
Virgin olive oil and vinegar	Butter or margarine
Pomegranate juice with sparkling water	Soda

Assignment #2: Kick Your Smoking Habit

If you smoke, quitting is a cornerstone of making yourself Heart Attack Proof. Not everyone can quit smoking in one week, but in this first week, commit to quit! Make a promise to yourself and your loved ones.

If you don't smoke or have already quit, congratulations! You are making one of the best decisions you can to protect your heart and your life. Why?

Smokers are two to three times more likely to die from coronary heart disease than nonsmokers. Smoking just one to four cigarettes per day equates to an almost three times higher risk of dying from coronary heart disease compared with not smoking. And each additional cigarette you smoke per day increases your risk.

Once you quit, your risk of heart disease and stroke will decrease no matter how long or how much you have smoked over your lifetime—even if you've been a heavy smoker! In fact, studies show that your cardiovascular risk will significantly decrease within the first two years of smoking cessation.

SMOKELESS TOBACCO USERS BEWARE: CAN YOUR CAN!

So you don't smoke cigarettes. Good. But if you use smokeless tobacco products like snuff and chewing tobacco, thinking they are healthier than lighting up—think again. Multiple studies conducted over the last thirty years have shown the opposite. Professors at the International Agency for Cancer Research in France analyzed data from over eleven studies conducted in Europe and North America and found that smokeless tobacco also greatly increases your risk of dying from a heart attack or stroke.

The same is true of your risk of dying from a heart attack—even if you have already suffered one! Israeli Professor Yaacov Drory recently examined this in his research published in *The Journal of the American College of Cardiology*. Professor Drory's data spanned more than thirteen years, and what he found was that quitting smoking after a heart attack, just on its own, was almost as effective as other approaches, including invasive procedures and statins or lipid-lowering drugs. He found that quitting smoking was the most important risk factor modification linked to long-term survival even after accounting for lifestyle, socioeconomics, and other cardiovascular risk factors (like lack of regular exercise and obesity). Compared to patients who continued to smoke, those who quit smoking before their first heart attack had a 50 percent lower mortality rate. And those who quit *after* their first heart attack still benefited: they lowered their risk by 37 percent.

Make this week the first week of your smoke-free life. No, it's not always easy. But the good news is that there are many new and better ways to help you quit, such as behavioral therapy and medication. Discuss smoking cessation options with your personal physician.

Some smoking cessation tips:

- If you can quit "cold turkey," do so. If not, smoke fewer and fewer cigarettes each day, until you can wean yourself off completely.
- Carry sugarless gum, and munch on healthy finger-food snacks like carrots, celery, and apple wedges to allay your cravings.
- Stay busy, manage your stress (see Week 3), and drink lots of water.
- Begin a regular walking program (see Week 2).
- Know your triggers! They are often why earnest attempts to quit fail.
- Don't beat yourself up. Stay positive. You *will* succeed.

For my patients, a combination of medication and socially supportive counseling has always seemed to work best. One great place to start is the Internet. There are many web-based support groups, including smokefree.gov, that can help get you on your path to a smoke-free life.

Your health insurance company also is a great resource. Many plans will cover the cost of counseling and medications to quit smoking.

Assignment #3: Check In for a Checkup

Understanding your current state of health is essential to achieving wellness and becoming Heart Attack Proof. The easiest way to do this is to pick up the phone, call your personal physician, and schedule an appointment for a routine evaluation. Here's why.

Reconnecting with your physician is always smart, especially when you are embarking on a new program, so that he or she will be aware of the changes you are making, can offer support and guidance, and can answer any questions you may have. For example, Week 2 is the week to start moving...as in exercising. And while your goal is just to start incorporating walks or bike rides into every week, it's good for your physician to be aware of this. Your healthcare provider may want to schedule you for a stress test prior to starting an exercise program—something that is especially important if you have risk factors for coronary heart disease, such as high cholesterol, high blood pressure, and/or diabetes, or have a history of heart disease.

As part of your routine evaluation, your doctor should perform a blood test, which is crucial to assessing your overall health, including your cardiovascular health. It's important for you to be aware of the new advanced blood tests that go beyond measuring standard cholesterol levels to uncover hidden risks for heart attack and stroke.

I've included a list of routine and additional cardiovascular tests you should request here. We'll talk more about them, specifically what they measure and why they're important, once you have the results, in Week 5.

Recommended Blood Tests

ROUTINE BLOOD TESTS

CBC (complete blood count)

Measures red and white blood cell, platelet, hemoglobin, and hematocrit levels in the blood

Why it's important: Red blood cells carry oxygen to all the cells in your body, and white blood cells play an important immune function. Platelet count is also important, since a low count can lead to bleeding and a high count can lead to thrombosis or clotting.

Chemistry panel

Assesses factors in the blood, including blood glucose (sugar); electrolytes such as calcium, potassium, and sodium; blood urea nitrogen and creatinine (which reflect kidney function); and transaminase levels and bilirubin (which reflect liver function)

Why it's important: A chemistry panel can reveal the presence or absence of a wide variety of disorders, such as diabetes, kidney or liver impairment, or electrolyte disturbance. All of these metabolic derangements can impact heart and vascular function and increase the risk of heart attack and stroke.

Thyroid function panel

Measures TSH (thyroid stimulating hormone), T4, and T3 in the blood

Why it's important: Thyroid disorders can have an impact on your heart. Low thyroid levels can raise cholesterol levels, and elevated thyroid levels can lead to palpitations and cardiac arrhythmias, such as atrial fibrillation.

Lipid profile

Assesses the total cholesterol, LDL (bad) cholesterol, HDL (good) cholesterol, and triglyceride levels in the blood

Why it's important: An elevated LDL cholesterol or a reduced HDL cholesterol increases the risk of heart attack. Recent studies have demonstrated that an elevated nonfasting triglyceride level also increases heart attack risk.

ADVANCED CARDIOVASCULAR BLOOD TESTS

hs-CRP

Measures high-sensitivity (hs) C-reactive protein in the blood

Why it's important: hs-CRP is a marker of vascular inflammation, and an elevated level is associated with an increased risk of heart attack and stroke.

Lp-PLA2

Measures Lp-PLA2 in the blood

Why it's important: LpPLA2 is associated with an increased risk of heart attack and stroke, and is an even more specific measurement of vascular inflammation than hs-CRP. Studies have shown that measurement of both hs-CRP and Lp-PLA2 is more predictive of heart attack and stroke risk than either test individually.

Myeloperoxidase

Measures myeloperoxidase in the blood

Why it's important: Myeloperoxidase is a marker of free radicals and oxidative stress. Elevated levels increase the risk of plaque instability and increase heart attack risk twofold.

ApoB

Measures the total number of (bad) cholesterol-carrying particles in the blood

Why it's important: apoB particles can enter the artery wall and lead to an atherosclerotic plaque. High levels of apoB have been shown to be a better predictor of heart attack risk than either total cholesterol or LDL cholesterol.

ApoA1

Measures the total number of cholesterol-carrying HDL (good) particles in the blood (every HDL particle carries an apoA1 molecule)

Why it's important: HDL particles can remove cholesterol from the artery wall and lead to a decrease in the size of atherosclerotic plaques. High levels of apoA1 are associated with a lower risk of heart attack.

ApoB : ApoA1 ratio

Measures the ratio of bad cholesterol–carrying particles to good cholesterol–carrying HDL particles in the blood

Why it's important: The ApoB : ApoA1 ratio has been shown to be one of the best predictors of future heart attack risk.

LDL-P

Measures the number of LDL cholesterol particles in the blood

Why it's important: Ninety percent of the atherogenic (bad) particles that enter the artery wall are LDL particles. Like apoB, LDL-P has also shown to be a better predictor of heart attack risk than total cholesterol or LDL-cholesterol.

Particle size

Measures the size of lipoprotein particles, such as LDL and HDL particles

Why it's important: Although particle number is more important than particle size, knowing the size of particles is still worthwhile. Small LDL particles have an easier time entering the artery wall and becoming trapped and oxidized (leading to atherosclerotic plaque development) than large LDL particles. Increased concentration of small LDL particles is also reflective of insulin resistance and diabetes as well as metabolic syndrome. The Quebec Cardiovascular Study found that an increased number of small particles raised heart attack risk sixfold, whereas an increased number of large particles raised risk twofold. In addition, HDL particle size can be informative, because large HDL particles are more efficient than small HDL particles in removing cholesterol from the artery wall.

LPa

Measures the amount of lipoprotein(a) in the blood

Why it's important: Lipoprotein-a (LPa) is an LDL particle with an attachment called apo-a. Elevated levels of LPa increase the risk of heart attack and stroke.

Omega-3 index

Measures the percentage of omega-3 fat in the red blood cell membrane

Why it's important: Low levels of omega-3 are associated with an increased risk of heart attack and an increased risk of sudden cardiac death. This increased risk can be lowered by raising omega-3 levels with diet (especially cold-water fish) or supplements.

Vitamin D

Measures the level of vitamin D in the blood

Why it's important: Low levels of vitamin D predict an increased risk of heart attack. A study by Dr Tami L Bair and colleagues (Intermountain Medical Center Heart Institute, Murray, Utah) presented at the American College of Cardiology 2010 Scientific Sessions concluded that correcting vitamin D deficiency can lower heart attack risk.

Assignment #4: Get a Dental Evaluation

You've got your doctor's appointment set up, but don't stop there! It's very important that you also make an appointment with a dentist for a thorough cleaning and checkup.

Your oral health can directly impact your heart health. Inflammation in your gums from periodontal disease increases the risk of cardiovascular disease. When your gums become infected, the bacteria in the affected periodontal tissue causes a generalized inflammatory response that increases the risk of heart attack and stroke.

Brushing and flossing your teeth regularly is key to preventing dental plaque buildup and reducing gingivitis, which is the beginning of periodontal disease. Periodontal disease literally means infection and inflammation around the tooth, and it can affect one tooth or many. If you aren't brushing and flossing on a regular basis, small particles of food can get trapped between your teeth and gums and lead to infection and dental plaque formation. Your gums can become tender, red, and swollen, and can bleed following brushing. That inflammatory response, in which the body aggressively attacks the dental tissue and bone, results in receding gums and tooth loss.

Are You Ready?

A clinical research study that followed more than 100,000 people with no history of heart attack or stroke for an average of seven years found that those who had their teeth cleaned by a dentist or dental hygienist at least twice a year for two years had a 24 percent lower risk for heart attack and a 13 percent lower risk for stroke compared to those who never went to the dentist or only went once in two years. These findings were presented at the 2011 American Heart Association's annual meeting in Orlando, Florida.

There's more. A 2004 New York University and Centers for Disease Control (CDC) survey identified a link between periodontal disease and diabetes in almost three thousand patients. Dr. Sheila Strauss of NYU's Colleges of Dentistry and Nursing determined that 93 percent of participants with periodontal disease were considered to be at high risk for diabetes, compared to just 63 percent of those without periodontal disease.

WEEK 1

Putting It Into Practice

This week your goal is to lay the foundation for the next five weeks by addressing several important factors of a Heart Attack Proof life. You should:

☐ Assess your food choices and become a traditional Mediterranean

☐ Commit to stop smoking

☐ See your doctor to get a complete physical exam and comprehensive blood test

☐ Visit your dentist for a checkup and cleaning

Week 2

Get Fit for Life

Lack of activity destroys the good condition
of every human being, while movement and
methodical physical exercise save it and preserve it.

—PLATO

HOW FAMILIAR IS THIS SCENARIO? You're sitting in the living room, and the phone starts ringing on the other side of the house. You sprint to pick it up in time, which leaves you needing a few moments to catch your breath and hoping that the person you've just said hello to can't tell that you're panting.

In the thirty seconds it probably took you to dash from the living room to the phone, your heart and body performed several functions. Your brain told your muscles that you needed to move, and quickly. Your lungs started expanding to increase the amount of oxygen you consumed, and your respiratory rate increased. Your heart went into overdrive to supply extra blood and oxygen to your muscles and get them moving.

While sprinting to answer the phone can't be considered strenuous exercise, in some ways, it is a mini-fitness test. *Fitness* has long been defined as the ability to perform daily tasks without fatigue or undue distress. But technological advances and a culture of efficiency have moved us from a life of daily functional activity to spending most of our time almost immobile on the couch. For all the strides we've made in the name of technological progress, we have taken two steps backward in health due to our sedentary lifestyle.

Exercise Is Essential

It's not that the technological advancements of our modern society are bad. We've certainly improved the quality of our lives and become a global society. From a medical standpoint, we have developed amazing tools and procedures to prolong and save lives. But we spend so much of our lives sitting—sitting at work toiling away at our computers, sitting at home in front of the television, sitting in our cars as we motor from place to place. Contrast that with the life of our hunter-gatherer ancestors, who relied on movement and activity for their very survival. The fact is, we are not genetically programmed to lead sedentary lives.

And viewed from an anatomical and physiological perspective, this inactivity is absolutely contrary to our makeup. The body is designed to move; we have over six hundred skeletal muscles designed to stretch, flex, bend, twist, jump, run, and more! Imagine a movement, and our bodies (when healthy) can likely do it. When many muscles are activated in larger groups, they stimulate blood circulation throughout the body and to all our organs, helping to remove toxins through sweating and other filtration methods, as well as improving the efficiency of our lungs and heart. It's no wonder that all of this physical inactivity is directly linked to poor health, specifically obesity, diabetes, heart attack, stroke, cancer, and more.

Truthfully, we've known how detrimental inactivity is for some time. Back in 1953, the British physician Dr. Jeremy Morris and his colleagues studied conductors working on London's double-decker buses. Morris compared the conductors, who climbed nearly six hundred stairs per workday, to bus drivers, who sat driving a bus for 90 percent of the day. He found that the conductors had half as many heart attacks as the bus drivers. Yet we live even more sedentary lives today than we did sixty years ago. What does this mean? It means that today we must make a conscious choice to be physically active. We can't depend on getting the amount of movement we require to live long, healthy lives in the course of our routine daily activities.

The "Heart" Truth

The truth is, exercise is essential to becoming Heart Attack Proof. There are no shortcuts, and to try to look for any would be depriving your mind, your body, and your heart of the amazing benefits of regular exercise.

That's because exercise really works. And not just for the young, fit, or accomplished. Study after study has shown that your body reaps the benefits of exercise, no matter what your age, weight, or proficiency level—even after only one session! It's so effective that the Institute of Medicine has recommended that physicians start prescribing exercise instead of, or in combination with, certain medications for a variety of conditions. Sound crazy? It's not.

Take a recent study of a high-risk group: elderly patients ages sixty-five to eighty-three with controlled type-2 diabetes, high blood pressure, and high blood cholesterol. Definitely a high-risk population! Dr. Kenneth Madden, a geriatric specialist at the University of British Columbia, decided to see if three months of exercise could improve the stiffness and elasticity of participants' arteries. (Increased arterial stiffness is associated with adverse cardiac events like heart attack and stroke.) Participants either did nothing and remained sedentary, or exercised for one hour three times a week on treadmills or cycling machines with supervision. After three months, the exercisers had a 15 to 20 percent reduction in arterial stiffness—a clinically significant reduction that most cardiologists would agree offers important protection against future heart attacks.

Exercise and Hypertension

While we're on the topic of arteries and how exercise and regular movement can keep them flexible, let's talk about blood pressure. Blood pressure is the measure of the force of the blood against the artery wall as it moves through your body, pumped from your heart. When you have your blood pressure taken, you are given two numbers, read as one number over the other.

The top number is your *systolic* pressure—the pressure of the blood against the artery wall when your heart contracts. The bottom number is your *diastolic* pressure—the pressure of the blood against the artery wall when the heart relaxes between beats. A normal blood pressure is 120/80 mmHg or lower. If your blood pressure is chronically higher than 140/90 mmHg, you have a condition called hypertension, or high blood pressure.

Hypertension is extremely common today. Most of us know someone with hypertension; in fact, more than 50 million Americans deal with it on a daily basis. But we don't have to. It is usually

Hypertension can lead to:

- Heart attack
- Stroke
- Kidney failure
- Abdominal aortic aneurysm

preventable. The scientific literature shows that regular exercise decreases blood pressure in about 75 percent of all people with hypertension.

Exercise and Heart Attack

Regular exercise has a beneficial impact on cholesterol, triglycerides, blood sugar, blood pressure, and inflammation. In addition, it helps to control body weight and avoid being overweight or obese. All of this contributes to significant reduction in the risk of a heart attack.

Like the early study of the London bus drivers, data proving that regular exercise can prevent heart attacks goes back decades. In a pivotal 1980 study of nearly twenty thousand male Civil Service workers, half as many men who engaged in exercise in their leisure time suffered or died from heart attacks over an eight-year period, as compared with men who had little leisure-time activity. Remarkably, the protective effects of exercise persisted even when the researchers accounted for smoking, obesity, family history of coronary heart disease, and existing hypertension. To quote the 1980 study abstract published in the journal *Lancet*:

> Men who engaged in vigorous sports, keep fit, and the like during an initial survey in 1968–70 had an incidence of CHD in the

The cardiovascular benefits of regular exercise:

- Lowers body weight
- Improves lipid profile: Lowers triglycerides and LDL (bad) cholesterol particles, and raises HDL (good) cholesterol
- Lowers inflammation
- Lowers risk of blood clots
- Lowers stress hormones (e.g., adrenalin)
- Lowers blood pressure and heart rate
- Dilates the coronary arteries
- Improves collateral circulation

next 8½ years somewhat less than half that of their colleagues who recorded no vigorous exercise. The generality of the advantage suggests that vigorous exercise is a natural defense of the body, with a protective effect on the ageing heart against ischemia and its consequences.

Exercise is so powerful, it even helps people with existing heart disease, including those who have already had a heart attack. If you have survived a heart attack, there is strong evidence to show that if you start exercising now, you can greatly improve your chances of preventing future heart attacks, as well as surviving a second attack should one occur.

Exercise and Stroke

The term *stroke* describes any interruption of blood (and the oxygen and nutrients it carries) to the brain, typically from a blocked or ruptured blood vessel. It's an extremely debilitating and often fatal cardiovascular event: stroke is the third leading cause of death and the most common form of debilitating handicap for adults. According to the National Stroke Association, someone has a stroke about every forty-five seconds, with women suffering strokes more often than men.

The risk factors for a "brain attack" are similar to those for a heart attack, including smoking, high blood pressure, and diabetes. And recovering from a stroke takes months or even years of rehabilitation, often without a full recovery.

Renowned epidemiologist and physician Dr. Charles Hennekens and his colleagues at Harvard looked at whether exercise protected male physicians against stroke. The study followed more than twenty thousand physicians for almost twelve years. Dr. Hennekens found that exercise vigorous enough to work up a sweat, even just once per week, decreased the risk of stroke by 26 percent.

Research studies have demonstrated that once an exercise routine is started, blood pressure, lipids (triglyceride and cholesterol), blood sugar, and inflammation improve, and the risk of heart attack is reduced.

Researchers have also been able to establish a relationship between the amount of exercise, measured in calories burned per week, and the degree of cardiovascular risk reduction. Even patients who have already suffered a heart attack and started exercising survive longer than their non-exercising counterparts. Expending between seven hundred and two thousand extra calories a week through exercising provides the greatest protective effect, especially in those who mainly have been sedentary.

Fit or Fat?

Clinical studies have shown that your physical activity level is a better predictor of a heart attack or adverse cardiac event than your body weight. Take professional football players. They have muscle, but many also have excess fat. So how healthy are they? Are they protected from heart disease?

Researchers at the University of Texas Southwestern Medical Center put those questions to the test with former National Football League players. What the researchers found was that all that fitness, regardless of the player's body fat, had paid off. The former footballers were better protected against heart disease compared to sedentary men their age, despite the fact that most NFL players have a body mass index (BMI) that categorizes them as overweight or obese. The findings, which were published in the *American Journal of Cardiology*, showed that the retired NFL players had a significantly lower prevalence of diabetes, hypertension, and metabolic syndrome compared to their nonathletic peers.

What this means is that it's more important to be fit and active, even if you're a bit overweight, than to have a normal body weight and be unfit. This isn't to say that we shouldn't strive to achieve an ideal body weight and a normal BMI (see Appendix A). It does, however, stress the importance of achieving fitness *as well as* normal body weight for optimum health.

Fat isn't evil; we all need to store some of it so we have an energy source for bodily functions when we deplete our primary energy source, glucose, a simple form of sugar. But not all fat is created equal. Research has shown that *visceral fat*—the fat that resides in the abdominal cavity and around internal organs—is particularly associated with health risks.

Research also shows that exercise helps keep off visceral fat. Exercise physiologists at the University of Alabama at Birmingham (UAB) found that as little as eighty minutes a week of aerobic or resistance training not only prevented weight gain in general, but also inhibited a regain of harmful visceral fat one year after weight loss.

In the study, which was published in the journal *Obesity*, UAB exercise physiologist Gary Hunter, PhD, and his team randomly assigned ninety-seven women to three groups: aerobic training, resistance training, or no exercise. (All had a restricted diet.) After the participants lost weight, researchers recorded the women's total fat, abdominal subcutaneous fat, and visceral fat. Participants in the two exercise groups were then asked to continue exercising forty minutes twice a week for one year. What the researchers found was that participants who continued exercising, despite slight overall weight gains, regained 0 percent of the visceral fat, compared to a 33 percent regain of visceral fat for those who stopped exercising or didn't exercise at all. And all of that from just two exercise sessions per week, a relatively small commitment!

EXERCISE IS MEDICINE

In 2007, the American Medical Association and the American College of Sports Medicine (ACSM) launched the "Exercise Is Medicine" program to advocate and encourage doctors to prescribe exercise to their patients as treatment. According to a recent ACSM survey, nearly two-thirds of patients said they would be more interested in exercising to stay healthy if advised to do so by their doctor.

Even More Benefits

You'll also see other perks from regular exercise beyond cardiovascular health. I'm sure you've heard of a runner's high. Joggers, runners, and walkers often describe this phenomenon, which is a state of euphoria experienced due to exercise. It's not all in their heads: aerobic activity produces a release of endorphins in the brain, leaving you feeling happy.

Exercise helps beat depression the same way, and it has been shown to be an effective way to treat anxiety, with similar or better results as compared to traditional medicinal therapy.

If you have decided to quit smoking, exercise can help, especially in combination with nicotine replacement therapies. And there are plenty of other documented benefits, from improved sleep quality to lower risk of cancer.

Additional benefits of exercise beyond heart health:

- Decreases anxiety and depression
- Reduces cravings to smoke
- Improves lung function
- Improves arthritis
- Improves sleep quality
- Improves memory
- Reduces signs of aging
- Improves bone health
- Lowers risk of cancer

Assignment: Get Moving!

This second week in your journey to become Heart Attack Proof is all about *moving*. Your task is to get moving and be consistent.

During this week, you will take your first steps toward a more active lifestyle, so if you don't have any favorite physical activities, now is a great time to try a few. Research shows that we are more likely to create fitness habits when we participate in activities we enjoy, which makes sense.

Where to Start?

You don't have to run a marathon to be fit. What is most important is that you exercise regularly.

Beginning your fitness routine is simple. Aside from picking the activity or activities you enjoy the most, there are three concepts to consider when planning your program:

- how often you plan to exercise (frequency)
- how hard you should exercise (intensity)
- how long you are able to exercise (time or duration)

To help you remember, the American Heart Association (AHA) created the "FIT Formula": *frequency*, *intensity*, *time*.

Wondering what exercise *frequency* and *time* will most benefit your heart, lungs, and circulation? Organizations like the AHA and the American College of Sports Medicine (ACSM) jointly recommend doing moderately intense cardio activities for thirty minutes a day, five days a week. Of course, you may need to start slowly if you are currently sedentary; aiming for twenty minutes of exercise three to five times a week is a great goal for the first few weeks. Eventually, however, you should strive to do at least thirty minutes of aerobic activity every day.

GET FIT (FREQUENCY, INTENSITY, TIME)

Frequency: 3–5 times per week

Intensity: Break a sweat but able to carry on a conversation

Time: 20–30 minutes

When it comes to *intensity*, a simple rule of thumb is that you should break a sweat but still be able to carry on a conversation while working out.

Walk This Way

One easy way to get more active is with a walking program. Start going for a walk every morning, or instead of sitting on the couch at night, get up and walk in place for thirty minutes while watching your favorite show.

If you think you can't get a great workout from walking, think again! Recent research shows that moving at a moderately brisk pace for forty-five minutes three times per week at about 60 percent of your maximum heart rate significantly increases cardiorespiratory fitness and can decrease blood pressure, plasma triglyceride, cholesterol, and bad LDL cholesterol levels, while increasing good HDL cholesterol concentrations. Participants in the study also lost body weight and fat stores, and even decreased their waist size!

Researchers from Harvard Medical School looking at stroke risk studied almost forty thousand female health professionals. The findings, which were published in 2010 in *Stroke: Journal of the American Heart Association*, showed that women who walked two or more hours a week were significantly less likely to suffer a stroke than less-active women.

Ten Thousand Steps a Day—The Key to a Healthy Heart

Walking ten thousand steps each day is considered to be the equivalent of sixty minutes of moderate intensity exercise. However, most of us walk less than three thousand steps per day.

In a study led by Peter T. Katzmarzyk, PhD, of the Pennington Biomedical Research Center, published in the *American Journal of Preventive Medicine,* those who walk ten thousand steps or more each day reduce their odds of developing metabolic syndrome by 72 percent.

Research in the *British Medical Journal* suggests that building up to ten thousand steps a day can help control weight and may reduce diabetes risk. Of 592 middle-aged Australian adults, those who increased the number of steps they took during a five-year period, building up to ten thousand steps per day, had a lower body mass index, less belly fat, and better insulin sensitivity than their counterparts who did not walk as much. All this walking also helps to reduce the risk of obesity, diabetes, and heart disease.

To help you get to ten thousand steps, consider purchasing a pedometer (most cost less than $20) that measures the number of steps you take. It is worth the investment.

> Increase your steps per day by:
> - Taking stairs rather than elevators
> - Walking during your lunch break
> - Walking in place while watching TV
> - Scheduling a 30–45 minute walk each day

Resistance Training

Resistance training and muscle-strengthening exercises, also called *isometric exercise*, involve using our muscles to pull or push weight, including our own body weight.

Resistance training promotes lean muscle mass and maintains muscle tone, which may help to efficiently metabolize glucose. In women, research shows that resistance training maintains bone mineral density, helping to ward off osteoporosis. In addition, keeping good muscle tone helps you maintain a healthy weight—lean muscle burns more calories than fat, thereby increasing your resting metabolism.

What are some good things to use as you begin resistance training? Your own body weight, resistance bands or pulleys, free weights, medicine balls, or weight machines are all good options. And there is no need to overdo it. Doing eight different resistance exercises at ten to twelve repetitions each is sufficient.

If you are starting a resistance or weight-training program for the first time, consider working with a certified personal trainer, at least for a few sessions.

CAUTION

Always check with your personal physician prior to starting an exercise program. If you have a history of cardiovascular disease or cardiac risk factors, your doctor may want you to have a stress test prior to clearing you for exercise.

Are You Ready?

I recommend starting to implement your Heart Attack Proof fitness plan by walking for thirty to forty-five minutes per day. If you have the time to enjoy other activities, such as tennis, golf (walking from hole to hole, not driving a golf cart), swimming, or biking, then do it! Otherwise, walk, walk, walk—your heart will thank you.

ACTIVE LIVING

In 1997 the CDC began the Active Living Initiative, which aims to better understand how our environment can be improved to support more active lifestyles, and taps into the expertise of urban planners, architects, engineers, public health experts, and physicians. "Active living" incorporates physical activity into daily routines, such as walking to the store or biking to work. How active is *your* living?

Want more information or to get involved? Visit http://www .activelivingbydesign.org.

TIP

If you can't squeeze a continuous 30 minutes of exercise into your day, try breaking those 30 minutes up into three 10-minute intervals. Studies have shown that this has just as much impact on improving your cardiovascular fitness.

Sample Fitness Plan: Beginner

Monday	Tuesday	Wednesday	Thursday	Friday	Saturday	Sunday
Rest	Walk 30 min	Bike 30 min	Walk 30 min	Rest	Walk 30 min	Walk 30 min

Sample Fitness Plan: Intermediate

Monday	Tuesday	Wednesday	Thursday	Friday	Saturday	Sunday
Walk 30 to 45 min	Walk 30 to 45 min	Strength train (see sample plan)	Bike 30 to 45 min	Walk 30 to 45 min	Walk 30 to 45 min	Strength train (see sample plan)

Sample Fitness Plan: Strength/Resistance Training

Exercise	Reps	Muscle Group
Push-ups	10	Chest
Biceps curls	10	Biceps
Triceps curls	10	Triceps
Lunges	8–10 each leg	Quadriceps, hamstrings
Overhead press	10	Shoulders
Sit-ups	12	Abdominals
Rowing	10	Back
Calf raises	12 each leg	Gastrocnemius

WEEK 2

Putting It Into Practice

Last week you should have called your doctor and your dentist; hopefully you've seen at least one of them by now. If you smoke, you should be making progress toward quitting, and you should have started eating more foods from the Mediterranean diet.

This week you should:

☐ Get clearance to start an exercise program from your personal treating physician.

☐ Get a pedometer and strive to take ten thousand steps per day.

☐ Incorporate one to two sessions per week of resistance or weight training into your fitness routine.

Week 3

Create a Stress-Free Lifestyle

Tension is who you think you should be.
Relaxation is who you are.

—CHINESE PROVERB

THIS WEEK IS ALL ABOUT learning how to manage the inevitable stress that affects each of us every day of our lives. How you handle stress can mean the difference between life and death.

Are you a worrier? Do you have anxiety? Do you toss and turn at night? Do you have a short fuse? Or do you hold everything in as long as you can and then explode? Are you a perfectionist or a workaholic?

The goal of this week is to understand your stress type, identify your triggers, and learn new ways to manage your stress. By doing so, you will lessen the negative effects stress can have on your life, the lives of your loved ones, and your body, particularly your heart.

I have found in my practice—and even in the medical community—that too often we overlook stress as a risk factor for heart disease. This may be because each of us perceives stress and stressors differently. Thus, stress is hard to actually measure. But just because we can't measure it doesn't mean it doesn't exist. We all experience stress, from the small stuff we're not supposed to sweat, like traffic jams and getting the kids to practice on time, to the big stuff, like being laid off from your job or dealing with a divorce or the passing of a loved one. They're all part of the daily stress stew.

It's important to know that you are not alone in feeling stress. We all experience it. But along the way, some of us have learned skills that make it easier to handle.

The Stress Response

Your body's ability to perceive and react to stress is actually a good thing—it's an ancient, innate defense mechanism designed to keep you alive. Early man relied on a sudden surge of stress hormones to fight off or flee an imminent threat, like a saber-toothed tiger—this is the fight-or-flight response. The problem for modern man is that, while we thankfully don't face off with wild animals anymore, our hormonal responses don't see it that way.

That car that just cut you off, the looming deadline to get that report in by the end of the day, and the washer breaking down (and how to pay for it!) all evoke a stress response. And to our bodies, it may as well have been a lion, tiger, or bear attacking us—perhaps all three in one day.

While ancient man may have confronted one or two stressful events in a week, today we have twenty to thirty stressful stimuli per day that our brains can perceive as direct threats. Pink slips, financial stressors, and marital strain feel just as threatening as a ferocious tiger, and when stressors like these occur on a regular basis, that adaptive response that saved our ancestors' life itself becomes a threat.

The sad fact of modern living is that we are in a constant state of physiological stress, and that can have a deleterious effect on our hearts. Stress and anger increase the release of stress hormones, such as adrenaline and cortisol. These have the natural effects of increasing blood pressure, cholesterol, and blood sugar; causing the heartbeat to become rapid; and increasing the "stickiness" of our platelets, which raises the likelihood of a blood clot. How well you handle daily stress is key to keeping your stress hormones, and the stress response, under control.

Hot Reactors

The heat wave won't let up, you're late, and you're caught in a massive traffic jam. Sound familiar? Just as you see an opening in the next lane, a car zips in front of you. You slam on the brakes, lay on the horn, and spout off a wave of expletives. You're going nowhere; your car isn't moving, much less your legs. But your heart is in overdrive! The stress on your heart is like driving eighty miles per hour with the brakes on. How much can your heart take before it says enough?

About forty years ago, cardiologist Dr. Robert Eliot did some groundbreaking research, finding that people who become angered easily in response to stressful situations also have extreme cardiovascular responses—their bodies produce large amounts of stress hormones and experience rapid rises in blood pressure and heart rate. These so-called "Hot Reactors" are quick to react to everyday stimuli, causing the stress response to happen multiple times a day, and are at greater risk for developing stress-related cardiovascular conditions such as heart attack and sudden cardiac death.

Hot Reactors are different from "Type A" personalities, workaholic types who are driven, competitive, impatient, and highly

HOT REACTOR QUIZ

- Do you get angry often?
- Do you experience chronic hostility?
- Do you explode when confronted with stress?
- Do you get red in the face and feel your heart pounding at even the slightest provocation?

If you answered yes to any of the above, you may be a Hot Reactor.

---

demanding of themselves and others. What we've learned is that, contrary to previous belief, being driven and ambitious does not increase the risk of suffering an adverse cardiac event. What really affects us is if we are habitually hostile and angry, because these traits activate a physical stress response through the sympathetic nervous system.

If you feel that you might be a Hot Reactor, discuss it with your healthcare provider, as there are ways to diagnose this condition. The good news is that Hot Reactors can be successfully treated with behavioral therapy and/or medication.

Anxiety

Chronic anxiety is also associated with negative cardiovascular outcomes. In a recent report published in the *Archives of General Psychiatry*, generalized anxiety disorder was associated with a 74 percent increased risk of a cardiovascular event in patients with coronary artery disease. So anxiety is something else you need to be aware of and manage.

Panic Attacks

Anxiety affects us all at different times and for different reasons. Job loss, fear of financial instability, life changes, and even small daily events can trigger feelings of helplessness or worry. For some, this may take the shape of a panic attack. Sufferers of panic attacks often described the experience as having an intense feeling of emergency, coupled with an inability to respond.

Physical symptoms of a panic attack can include extreme shortness of breath, rapid heartbeat, chest pain, and a feeling of impending doom. Some attacks are so bad that they prevent sufferers from going out, being social, or participating in any activity that could trigger the anxiety.

Clinical studies have shown that panic attacks, like general chronic anxiety, may be linked to a higher risk of a heart attack. Researchers at the University College London looked at data from more than 300,000 individuals and found that people diagnosed with panic attacks are 33 percent more likely to have a heart attack than those without the condition. In addition, heart disease among study participants with panic symptoms was especially high among women under fifty. The study, published in the *European Heart Journal*, stressed the need to discuss any panic attack symptoms with your healthcare provider. If you are prone to panic attacks, or have had them in the past, it is important that your personal physician is aware of them, as they can be managed through behavioral therapy and with medication.

Distressed and Depressed

Fred was a recently divorced father of two teenage boys. He was in his early fifties, and had led a relatively healthy, low-stress life. He was active, volunteered in his community, and had a long, successful career in advertising. Then the economy took a downturn, and Fred lost his job. Naturally, he began worrying about how he would take care of his boys, and where he would find the money for them to go to college. Fred started to become depressed.

The first time I met Fred was in the hospital, after he had suffered a heart attack. He told me how after he lost his job he slowly stopped communicating with his friends. He lost touch with his former colleagues, many of whom tried numerous times to reach out to him. He was tired and didn't have the energy to volunteer. And after unsuccessfully vying for several new positions, he felt defeated, old, inadequate, and worthless.

Fred is an example of an isolated, depressed individual. These people are the opposite of the Type A and Hot Reactor types, but are also at a greater risk for heart disease and sudden cardiac arrest than those who maintain strong support networks and social circles.

This personality has recently been given a name: Type D— Distressed and Depressed. Type Ds are characterized as identifying with chronic negative emotions, pessimism, and social inhibition.

Researchers at the University of Tilburg in the Netherlands looked at forty-nine studies of more than six thousand Type D patients with heart conditions to assess their future heart health. What they found was that the chronically down and isolated person was three times more likely to suffer a future cardiovascular event, including heart attack or sudden cardiac death, than a non–Type D person.

A Type D profile was also linked to a threefold increase in long-term risk of psychological conditions, including clinical depression, anxiety, and poor mental health. "Type D patients tend to experience increased levels of anxiety, irritation and depressed mood over time, while not sharing these emotions with others because of fear of disapproval," noted Viola Spek, PhD, a researcher and author of the study, which was published in the American Heart Association journal *Circulation*. "We found that a Type D personality predicts mortality and morbidity in these patients, independent of traditional medical risk factors."

In another study, the National Heart, Lung and Blood Institute and researchers at Indiana University-Purdue University Indianapolis examined the relationship between depression and inflammation in the body. They found that, over time, depressive symptoms are associated with increases in interleukin-6 (IL-6), an inflammatory protein that can predict cardiovascular events.

According to the study, which was published in the journal *Brain, Behavior and Immunity*, the relationship between depression and future heart disease is similar in strength to well-known risk factors like smoking, high blood pressure, and elevated cholesterol.

If you find you are more of a Type D personality than Type A, managing stress for you will mean learning to reach out to friends and family more, trying to meet new people and try new things, and generally staying upbeat and active. And remember, exercise, even moderate walking, has been proven to increase the release of endorphins, the "feel-good" hormones, as well as alleviating depression.

Managing depression is vital to your survival, especially if you already have underlying heart disease, according to a recent study of approximately six thousand British citizens who were followed for more than five years. Researchers from Europe and the United States determined that patients with heart disease and depression were five times more likely to die of any cause than those patients with only depression or only heart disease. So if you suffer from depression, discuss it with your physician, and get evaluated and treated by a qualified mental health professional.

Assignment: Learn to Manage Your Stress

We all have a little Hot Reactor in us and we all understand feelings of anxiety. Minimizing both will boost your happiness quotient and help you mentally and physically. No matter who you are, you will benefit from techniques and methods—from meditation and yoga to simply laughing more—to manage your stress, lighten your load, and live a happier and healthier life.

Practice the Relaxation Response

Your mental state is different than your physical state. This means you can retrain your mind to see daily stressors for what they are and not as ferocious beasts. Put more simply: you can learn to calm yourself down. One of the easiest and simplest things you can do the very first moment of panic or anxiety is to try to start breathing deeply and slowly. In contrast to the stress response, deep breathing calms the body and lowers heart rate and blood pressure. It's one of the most important processes in the body's relaxation response.

Many years ago, Dr. Herbert Benson of Harvard Medical School, founder of the Mind-Body Institute in Boston, shared with me a revolutionary way to manage stress. He identified the steps in the body's natural relaxation response and put them into deliberate practice. Today I recommend this simple process to all of my patients. It only takes ten to twenty minutes, and it does wonders for minimizing stress and your body's response to it.

Breathing is also a key component of many other relaxation techniques, including meditation, yoga, and even exercise.

THE RELAXATION RESPONSE

The relaxation response is a wonderful tool you can use to manage your stress, any time and almost anywhere.

1. Sit quietly in a comfortable position.
2. Close your eyes and visualize each of your muscles relaxing, beginning with your feet, moving up through your thighs, up to your back, through your neck, arms, and hands, and up to your face. Release any tension, and let your muscles remain relaxed.
3. Breathe deeply and slowly throughout this process. Focus your attention to your breathing and how your chest rises and falls with each inhale and exhale.
4. When you are comfortable, choose a word that represents relaxation to you (perhaps something like *peace* or *calm*). Silently repeat it to yourself with each inhalation.
5. Continue for about ten minutes, or as long as you feel comfortable.
6. Once your relaxation is complete, allow yourself to sit quietly for several more minutes, reawakening your senses a bit at a time. Don't feel pressure to stand until you are alert.

Meditation

Some think mediation is too alternative or too existential, but it can really be whatever you want it to be. The techniques of meditation can be traced back more than five thousand years. Meditation is actually very similar to the relaxation response. It just adds imagery, additional words or sayings, sounds, or symbols. The purpose of meditation is to allow the body to relax and the mind to focus on something positive.

Meditation also has a positive effect on the cardiovascular system. One type of meditation you may have heard of is *transcendental meditation*, which involves closed eyes and the use of a mantra or specific saying. In a study of two hundred patients with coronary heart disease, those who practiced transcendental meditation for twenty minutes twice per day had an almost 50 percent lower rate of heart attack, stroke, and death compared to non-meditating patients.

Beyond cardiovascular health, meditation:

- improves the ability to manage pain
- reduces anger and hostility
- enhances cognitive abilities
- increases attention span

Blood pressure can also be lowered through meditation. A study at the Medical College of Wisconsin found that participants who engaged in meditation not only decreased their blood pressure, but also perceived their stress levels to be lower.

You don't have to practice transcendental meditation to achieve these results. You just need to incorporate relaxation time in your day, using whatever technique you like most.

Yoga

Meditation is often included as part of yoga, another Eastern discipline that can be traced back some five thousand years. Simply translated as "union," yoga connects the body with the spirit in order to achieve peace, physical and mental balance, and well-being. In the last few years, yoga has become extremely popular, shifting in public perception from an alternative type of exercise to one that is offered at almost every gym in the country, not to mention the countless yoga-specific studios. Today yoga is practiced by all types of people from all age groups and backgrounds. Anyone seeking a stress-free life, from moms busy with kids to professional athletes, can appreciate the benefits of yoga.

Relying on deep breathing as the foundation of its practice, yoga is based on hundreds of poses, or *asanas*, each designed to promote relaxation, balance, flexibility, and strength. Because yoga is noncompetitive, it promotes self-acceptance and stresses concentration and listening to your body and mind.

Yoga has been shown to improve many disorders, from depression and anxiety, to pain and asthma, to, yes, cardiovascular issues. In the journal *Psychosomatic Medicine*, Ohio State University researchers recently reported results from a study showing that women who routinely practiced yoga had lower amounts of the inflammatory marker interleukin-6 (IL-6) in their blood than nonpracticing women. The practicing women also showed smaller increases in IL-6 after stressful experiences than women of the same age and weight who were not yoga practitioners. IL-6, as you may recall from Week 1, is an important part of the body's inflammatory response and has been shown to be a biomarker in heart disease, stroke, type-2 diabetes, arthritis, and other inflammatory and age-related diseases.

The study also measured C-reactive protein (CRP), another key inflammatory marker, which was discussed in Week 1 as part of your comprehensive blood test. The researchers found that women who did not practice yoga had CRP levels 4.75 times higher than women who regularly engaged in the mind-body exercise.

Another study out of Boston University's School of Medicine identified that a yoga session increased levels of gamma-aminobutyric acid (GABA), a chemical that is reduced in people with mood and anxiety disorders. The researchers reported that increased GABA levels after a yoga session were associated with improved mood and decreased anxiety, more so than the increases seen after moderate exercise.

Asanas for Stress

One of the easiest ways to experience yoga and begin to incorporate it into your life is to take a class. If you belong to a gym, check to see if they have yoga instruction; typical class names include Yoga Flow, Vinyasa Yoga, Hatha Yoga, and the like. Because yoga is noncompetitive, almost all classes welcome beginners, except classes like Power Yoga, which are designed for those with considerable strength and cardiovascular fitness. As with any new physical activity, be sure to check with your doctor before starting.

Take a Nap

Many people say we don't have time for naps. However, if you do not get enough sleep, it can feel like you are sitting on a large pile of explosives: you're often short-tempered and more vulnerable to stress.

Clinical studies support the benefits of a midday nap. The Harvard School of Public Health in Boston studied more than 23,000 Greek adults and published the results in the *Archives of Internal Medicine*. They found that people who regularly took a nap—a common practice in many of the Mediterranean countries—were more than 30 percent less likely to die of heart disease. "Taking a nap could turn out to be an important weapon in the fight against coronary mortality," said Dimitrios Trichopoulos, who led the study.

It is natural to feel drowsy in the afternoon, and many adults understandably experience a decrease in alertness after six to eight hours of working, especially if they don't get enough sleep at night. But for some reason our culture frowns on the idea of midday naps for anyone other than small children or the elderly.

The truth is, napping can provide significant health benefits. Research has shown that a brief nap can result in greater alertness, reduced levels of stress, and improved cognitive function. Napping also improves mental and cognitive abilities. A NASA study showed that a short nap boosted airline pilots' performance by 33 percent. In fact, a midday catnap can recharge your batteries better than drinking a cup of coffee: studies show that people who power nap get better results on memory tests than those who drink caffeine.

What's a *power nap*? A fifteen- to thirty-minute snooze. Be careful not to sleep too long: most experts feel that napping more than thirty minutes in the afternoon makes it more difficult for you to fall asleep at night.

Get More Nighttime Sleep

Sleep quality and quantity affects your risks of disease, including diabetes and heart disease. And data coming out of the West Virginia University School of Medicine is pointing to a direct relationship between sleep time—whether too short or too long—and cardiovascular disease.

When researchers looked at the sleep patterns and other demographic and lifestyle characteristics of 30,397 adults who participated in the 2005 National Health Interview Survey, they found that people who reported sleeping less than five hours per night were twice as likely to develop cardiovascular disease as those who slept seven hours. Interestingly, those who slept nine hours or more also had an increased risk of developing cardiovascular disease, even after accounting for factors that might otherwise influence the results. So while everyone's different, most of us should aim to sleep seven to eight hours a night.

According to the authors of the study, which was published in the journal *SLEEP*, the mechanisms underlying the association between short sleep and cardiovascular disease may include sleep-related disturbances in endocrine and metabolic functions, such as impaired glucose tolerance, reduced insulin sensitivity, increased sympathetic activity, and elevated blood pressure, all of which increase the risk of heart attack and stroke.

Similarly, researchers from the University of Warwick and the State University of New York at Buffalo discovered that people who sleep less than six hours per night may be three times more likely to find themselves in a pre-diabetic state between meals called *impaired fasting glucose*, or IFG. People with impaired fasting glucose are typically at a greater risk for developing type-2 diabetes. Men and women with insulin resistance and impaired fasting glucose, as well as those with diabetes, have an increased risk of heart attack and stroke.

A similar study published in the *Journal of Clinical Endocrinology & Metabolism* looked at sleep loss and insulin resistance in healthy people. What researchers at the Leiden University Medical Center in the Netherlands found was alarming: just one night of sleeping only four hours induced a temporary state of insulin resistance in healthy adults.

Finally, inadequate sleep has also been associated with increased consumption of sweet and fatty foods due to an increase in the body of the hunger hormone ghrelin, which means that not getting enough sleep could also contribute to weight gain.

Sleep Apnea—A New Risk Factor for Heart Attack

The nighttime breathing disorder known as *obstructive sleep apnea* increases a person's risk of having a heart attack or dying by 30 percent over a period of five years, according to a recent study. The study found that the more severe the sleep apnea, the greater the risk of developing heart disease or dying.

In obstructive sleep apnea, the upper airway narrows or collapses during sleep. Periods of apnea end with a brief partial arousal that can disrupt sleep hundreds of times a night. Because of these disruptions, sleep apnea triggers the fight-or-flight mechanism, which increases the risk of heart attack. In addition, episodes of apnea or breathing cessation results in decreased oxygen saturation in the bloodstream.

Yale University researcher Neomi Shah, MD, reported: "While previous studies have shown an association between sleep apnea and heart disease, ours is a large study that allowed us to not only follow patients for five years and look at the association between sleep apnea and the combined outcome of heart attack and death, but also adjust for other traditional risk factors for heart disease." Shah went on to say that "there is some evidence to make us believe that when sleep apnea is appropriately treated, the risk of heart disease can be lowered."

Risk factors for obstructive sleep apnea include:
• Family history of sleep apnea
• Use of alcohol, sedatives, or tranquilizers, which relax the muscles in your throat
• Overweight or obesity
• Neck circumference greater than 17 inches
• High blood pressure
• Diabetes
• Cigarette smoking
• Enlarged tonsils or adenoids, which narrow or block the airway
• Being male (men are twice as likely to have sleep apnea)
• Being over the age 65

The signs and symptoms of obstructive sleep apnea include periods of apnea (breathing cessation) during the night, snoring, daytime fatigue or drowsiness, irritability, morning headaches, and memory loss. The diagnosis of sleep apnea is made by conducting a formal sleep study. Treatment includes lifestyle changes, surgery, or nasal CPAP (continuous positive airway pressure). In CPAP, which has so far proven to be the most effective treatment, air is delivered through a mask while the patient sleeps, keeping the airway open. It has proven successful in many cases, providing a good night's sleep, preventing daytime accidents due to sleepiness, and improving quality of life.

If you have signs or symptoms of sleep apnea, notify your physician as soon as you can. Early recognition and management may lower your risk of a heart attack or stroke.

Spend Time With Friends

Social isolation can also wreak havoc on your heart. A study from the National Heart, Lung, and Blood Institute suggested that social isolation adversely impacts the cardiovascular system by activating the sympathetic nervous system and the hypothalamic-pituitary-adrenal pathways.

Other studies have analyzed the effects of isolation on elderly populations. Older men with few personal relationships have increased risk of heart disease, according to a report presented at the American Heart Association's Scientific Sessions 2003. And in a study examining factors that influence successful aging, researchers found that among a group of men in their seventies, social isolation was linked to increased levels of C-reactive protein (CRP), interleukin-6 (IL-6), and fibrinogen in the blood. These blood components are elevated during inflammation, and recent research has suggested that inflammation in the body is a risk marker for cardiovascular disease. People with elevated CRP and fibrinogen have higher risks for heart attack and stroke.

Laugh

One final note about managing your stress: there is simply nothing better for mood, stress release, the body, and overall well-being than a good, deep laugh. Children laugh an average of three hundred times per day. Adults? About fifteen times if we're lucky. It's important to remember how good it feels to laugh and how beneficial it can be to your health. Laughter may very well be the best medicine.

Anecdotally, I have noticed over the years that my patients who seemed to laugh more, take things in stride, and find a bit of humor in even the most stressful news had fewer heart attacks and lived longer. And I've come across study after study that identifies the ways that laughter promotes a beneficial, feel-good response in the body, and specifically improves cardiovascular health.

Laughter is particularly effective for stress management. According to Steve Sutanoff, PhD, a psychologist and the president of the American Association for Therapeutic Humor, "With deep, heartfelt laughter, it appears that serum cortisol, which is a hormone that is secreted when we're under stress, is decreased."

Laughter even seems to affect the blood vessels themselves. Research done at the cardiology department of Athens Medical School found that laughter improved arterial stiffness in healthy individuals. Similarly, studies at the University of Maryland Medical Center in Baltimore suggest that laughing may be as beneficial as exercise in relaxing arteries and increasing blood flow.

Some scientists have hypothesized that laughter releases chemicals that are protective to the artery lining, preventing cholesterol from entering the arterial wall to form the plaques that cause heart attack. Michael Miller, MD, director of the University of Maryland's Center for Preventive Cardiology, said, "Because we know many more factors that contribute to heart disease than factors that protect against it, the ability to laugh—either naturally or as a learned behavior—may have important implications in certain societies such as the United States, where heart disease remains the number one killer . . . Fifteen minutes of hearty laughter each day should be part of a healthy lifestyle."

Even the mere *expectation* of laughing, or seeing a comedic movie, or telling a funny joke, makes us feel good and can have a positive impact on our health. An interesting study split sixteen people into two groups. One group was told they would be watching a funny movie, and the other group was not. Blood was drawn

FACT

There are more than 6,000 laughter clubs in 60 countries!

from all subjects just before the video was started. The subjects who had been told they were going to see a funny movie had 27 percent more beta-endorphins (the feel-good hormone) in their blood sample than subjects in the other group. Furthermore, these beta-endorphin levels remained elevated during the video and for twelve to twenty-four hours afterward. It was concluded that these results, combined with other research on how laughter improves mood, are proof positive of just how good a hearty chuckle is for wellness, disease prevention, and stress reduction.

In Austria, "laughter yoga"—a mix of breathing, laughing, and stretching—has been shown to improve the recovery and well-being of stroke victims at Graz University, and may significantly lower blood pressure.

Who doesn't feel relaxed, calm, and happy after a good bout of laughter? Often in our stressful lives we forget to embrace the things we can do naturally to bring joy to ourselves and others. Laughing is a physiologic response, just like coughing or crying. We must remember to use it.

WEEK 3

Putting It Into Practice

You are halfway to becoming Heart Attack Proof! By Week 3, you've had a routine and thorough checkup with both your doctor and your dentist. You've had your blood drawn and sent out for a comprehensive analysis to evaluate your risk for heart attack and stroke. And with the help of family, friends, and your doctor, you've made the decision to stop smoking, started a Mediterranean-style diet, and gotten more physically active. You have an exercise plan in place and are working up a sweat three to four times per week, even if just by taking a walk with friends in the evening.

This week you should:

☐ Actively find ways to manage your stress.

☐ Practice the relaxation response.

☐ Share your cardiac makeover plans and successes with friends and family.

☐ Tell a joke, share a smile, and laugh!

Week 4

Achieve Optimal Nutrition

Let food be your medicine and medicine
be your food.

—HIPPOCRATES, 400 B.C.

THIS WEEK IS ALL ABOUT FOOD, and why what you eat matters. You wouldn't put the wrong fuel in your car, so why put the wrong food in your body? The toxic American or Western diet is highly processed, calorie dense, and nutrient depleted. But it doesn't just lead to obesity; it also seriously endangers your cardiovascular health.

This week, I'm going to make it easy for you to understand the importance of food choices. And then I will tell you what amazing, tasty foods are out there that will make you healthier and help you lose weight naturally without stress or struggle. They're the cornerstones to becoming Heart Attack Proof.

Are You Overweight?

In Week 1, you started making changes to your diet to eat more Mediterranean foods, and in Week 2, you started exercising more. If you've done both successfully, you may have noticed that you're already starting losing weight. But there may be more you need to do.

How much do you weigh? Do you feel it is optimal? Have you been carrying around an extra ten, twenty, or fifty pounds that you wish you could shed? Living with extra fat is a known risk factor not only for heart attack and stroke, but also for a multitude of other diseases, from diabetes to cancer to osteoarthritis.

Sometimes weight doesn't tell the entire story, however. That's why the medical community also relies on a metric called the Body Mass Index (BMI).

Body Mass Index (BMI)

When physicians and researchers discuss statistics on how many people in this country are overweight or obese, they are based on the BMI.

Your BMI is a measure of your body fat. It can be calculated by using this formula:

BMI (lbs / inches²) = (weight in pounds) x 703 ÷ (height in inches) x (height in inches)

Since this is a rather complicated formula, there are many online calculators to figure your BMI, and I also have provided a handy chart in Appendix A.

The benefit of the BMI is that it standardizes risk based on both height and weight. A BMI of 18.5 to 24.9 is considered normal, a BMI of 25 to 29.9 is overweight, and a BMI greater than 30 is obese.

More than 60 percent of the U.S. population is overweight or obese. That's right—almost two out of three people are at greater risk for cardiovascular disease and a number of other diseases based on their BMI.

> Besides increasing the risk of heart attack and stroke, obesity also increases the risk of:
> - Hypertension
> - Type-2 diabetes
> - Abnormal cholesterol and triglyceride levels
> - Cancer
> - Gallbladder disease
> - Sleep apnea syndrome
> - Osteoarthritis

A Family Problem

It's not just adults becoming bigger and heavier. Our children are also becoming overweight and obese at an alarming rate. According to the CDC, childhood obesity has tripled over the last thirty years, and presently one in three children in America is either overweight or obese.

Research shows alarming statistics about children with fatty streaks—the earliest stage of atherosclerosis, and a precursor to cardiovascular disease. In a sample population of five- to seventeen-year-olds, 70 percent of obese youth had at least one risk factor for cardiovascular disease.

Generally speaking, overweight and obese children will become overweight and obese adults, making them ticking time bombs for heart attacks. Luckily, the easiest time to change unhealthy habits

OUR CHILDREN AT RISK!

One-third of U.S. children are overweight or obese, putting them at higher risk of heart attack and stroke. Many experts predict that today's children will not live as long as their parents—the first time ever that an entire generation's life expectancy has dropped.

is at a young age. If you have children in your household, the lifestyle changes you make for yourself will likely positively affect them as well.

The Obesity Culprit—
The Toxic American Diet and Lifestyle

Most people are already well aware that obesity is far more common today than it was just a few decades ago. But did you know that the United States also has one of the highest rates of obesity in the world?

Part of the reason is what our typical American diet *doesn't* include: enough fresh fruit, vegetables, and whole grains. Instead, we have replaced these naturally available food sources with highly processed and convenient foods that lead to weight gain and damage our health.

Many of the processed foods that are widely available in our supermarkets, grocery stores, and fast-food restaurants have been stripped of their key healthful ingredients and pumped full of artificial preservatives. Moreover, our food contains excessive amounts of unhealthy fats, refined sugar, and sodium.

Fat: The Good, the Bad, and the Ugly

There are three types of fat in our diet: unsaturated fat (good), saturated fat (bad), and trans fat (just plain ugly).

Unsaturated fat, particularly polyunsaturated fat, is considered healthy. Polyunsaturated fats can have a beneficial effect on your health when consumed in moderation and when used to replace saturated fats or trans fats; they can help reduce the cholesterol levels in your blood and lower your risk of heart disease. They also include essential fats, such as omega-6 and omega-3, that your

KNOW YOUR FATS	
FAT TYPE	EXAMPLES
Unsaturated	Vegetable oil, fish oil
Saturated	Butter, meat, cheese
Trans fats	Packaged cookies, chips, pastries

body needs but can't produce. You must get these essential fats through the food you eat.

Saturated fats are unhealthy fats. They raise (bad) LDL cholesterol and increase the risk of heart disease and cancer. They are found in animal products, such as red meat, lard, butter, milk and cheese, and certain tropical oils, like palm and coconut oil.

Trans fatty acids, or trans fats, are even worse. They are manufactured fat borne out of an evolving need for more efficient foods that can withstand long shelf lives. Trans fats are created by taking oils—mainly vegetable oils—and putting them through a process called *hydrogenation*. Trans fats are found in many sweet,

CAUTION

Beware of hidden trans fats. Food companies are allowed to list zero trans fat on their label as long as the product contains 500 mg of trans fat or less per serving. This doesn't seem like much, but what if five of the items you eat each day have this amount? Now you are consuming 2,500 mg of trans fat in one day! The result is a significant amount of trans fat consumption by duped consumers who think they are eating healthy.

Since our own government doesn't protect us, we have to protect ourselves. Here's one of the easiest ways: if the ingredient summary on the label of the food you're thinking of purchasing lists partially hydrogenated oil, don't buy it!

Common foods that contain trans fat:

- Cake mixes
- Candy
- Chips
- Coffee creamers
- Cookies
- Crackers
- Doughnuts
- Margarine
- French fries
- Vegetable shortening

savory, and processed foods like margarine, French fries, potato chips, cookies, crackers, baked goods and pastries, and certain frozen foods—most of which can be stored for many months without going rancid. While scientists may have succeeded in making food last longer with trans fats, they couldn't have created something worse for our health. Trans fats raise (bad) LDL cholesterol, lower (good) HDL cholesterol, increase inflammation in the body, and make blood clots more likely to form.

Trans fat consumption has been linked to heart disease, cancer, Alzheimer's disease, and diabetes. It has been found to be so harmful that some health-conscious countries, like Denmark, have banned their use altogether. In America, states such as California have banned them from the restaurant food supply, as have certain cities, including New York City, Boston, and Philadelphia. Still, until America as a whole does the same, your best weapon against trans fat consumption is checking food labels—don't put trans fats in your body!

An easy way to avoid trans fat consumption is to avoid processed foods. I use what I call the "packaging test." Think about the foods you eat most often. How elaborate is the packaging? Is the food contained in a wrapper, like shrink-wrapped pastries or chips in a cardboard tube? If so, chances are the food is highly processed. (An exception: fruits and vegetables that are frozen and packaged right after they are picked.) Compare this to non-packaged whole foods, like a bunch of carrots or bananas.

CAUTION

All cooking oils—even "healthy" ones—contain a mixture of saturated and unsaturated fats. While some oils, such as olive oil, canola oil, and corn oil are considered healthier than others, it is recommended that all oils be used in moderation, since studies have demonstrated that excess consumption of cooking oils can be deleterious to your health and increase your risk for a heart attack. Let's also remember that oils are high caloric—a tablespoon is over one hundred calories. Therefore heed the old adage—drizzle, don't pour!

High-Fructose Corn Syrup

Most of us know to avoid excess sugar, whether in the form of table sugar or in candy or sweet syrups. But there's an even more sinister sweetener lurking on your shelves: high-fructose corn syrup. This is a favorite of the food industry, since it is sweeter than ordinary table sugar, is inexpensive, and prolongs the shelf life of a product. It is found in many beverages and foods, including soft drinks, sports drinks, packaged cookies, and other baked goods.

The real danger posed by high-fructose corn syrup and table sugar, however, is not the calories—it's the metabolic havoc they cause. Both of these sweeteners contain an equal amount of glucose and fructose. Fructose is not utilized by our muscles as an energy source; it goes directly to the liver, where it spikes triglyceride production, a major risk factor for heart disease.

And that's not all. New research presented at the American Society of Nephrology's 42nd Annual Meeting and Scientific Exposition in San Diego, California, showed that people who ate or drank more than seventy-four grams per day of fructose (the equivalent of only 2.5 soft drinks) increased their risk of developing high blood pressure or hypertension. A normal blood pressure reading is below

COINCIDENCE? HIGH-FRUCTOSE CORN SYRUP AND OBESITY

Since its introduction in 1970, the amount of high-fructose corn syrup in our food has steadily increased. Currently the average American consumes about 75 pounds of this sweetener each year. During the same time period, American obesity rate jumped from 15 to 30 percent. Many nutritionists believe this is no coincidence.

120/80 mmHg, but consuming more than seventy-four grams of fructose per day led to a 28 percent, 36 percent, and 87 percent higher risk for blood pressure levels of 135/85, 140/90, and 160/100 mmHg respectively, in a study population of 4,528 adults eighteen years of age or older with no prior history of hypertension.

While the controversy regarding high-fructose corn syrup continues, what isn't controversial is that excess consumption of sugar, in any form, should be avoided. What should you use instead? Many nutritionists believe that sweeteners derived from the stevia plant are preferable, since it is natural and low in calories.

The Beef With Beef

Most Americans eat too much red meat, and if you eat five ounces of red meat more than once a week, you are one of them. Research study after research study has shown that red meat is bad for our health, yet we skirt around the issue and downplay the serious health consequences of eating it. In this country, we are obsessed with red meat. We have bacon (yes, pork is a red meat) for breakfast, a hamburger or hot dog for lunch, and steak or meatloaf for dinner. Gourmet hamburger restaurants are the rage, and extensive commercial marketing campaigns have been launched to support red meat's continued consumption.

Years of scientific research have proven that this is dangerous eating. If you want a real cardiac makeover, one that will lead to a life without heart disease, and if you consume red meat on a regular basis, you will have to make seismic changes.

What's Wrong with Meat?

Red meat is high in saturated fats, which raise bad (LDL) cholesterol and increase the risk of atherosclerotic coronary heart disease. Red meat also is high in omega-6 fatty acids. Whereas omega-3 fatty acids, which are found in cold-water fish, help reduce inflammation in the body and have protective effects, omega-6 fatty acids actually promote inflammation.

Research has shown that red meat consumption is linked to:

- Cancer (colorectal, breast, prostate, and pancreatic)
- Chronic Inflammation
- Diabetes
- Elevated cholesterol
- Heart disease
- Hypertension

Findings from one of the largest studies ever, of more than 500,000 middle-aged and elderly Americans, were recently reported. The study looked at the dangers of meat consumption and its effect on dying prematurely and found that those who consumed four ounces of red meat a day (about the equivalent of a small hamburger) were more than 30 percent more likely to die during the ten years they were followed, mostly from heart disease and cancer. For this study, red meat included beef, pork, and all processed meat.

The study's lead author, Dr. Rashmi Sinha of the National Cancer Institute, stated, "The bottom line is we found an association between red meat and processed meat and an increased risk of mortality." In contrast, routine consumption of fish, chicken, and turkey decreased the risk of death by a small amount.

Barry M. Popkin, PhD, a professor of global nutrition at the University of North Carolina who wrote an editorial accompanying the study, added, "This is a slam-dunk to say that, 'Yes, indeed, if people want to be healthy and live longer, consume less red and processed meat.'"

Why is the consumption of red meat so unhealthy? There are many explanations:

- Cooking red meat generates cancer-causing compounds; red meat is also high in saturated fat, which has been associated with cardiovascular disease and various types of cancer.
- Meat is high in iron, which is also believed to promote cancer.
- Processed meats contain substances known as *nitrosamines*, which have been linked to cancer.
- People who eat red meat are more likely to have high blood pressure and elevated cholesterol, which increases the risk of heart disease.

New research continues to prove this point. The Harvard School of Public Health's Department of Nutrition looked at the effects of changing the proteins in women's diets, studying more than 84,000 women over a period of twenty-six years. Their results, published in *Circulation: Journal of the American Heart Association*, indicated that women who had two servings of red meat per day had a 30 percent greater risk of developing heart disease than women who opted for one-half of a serving per day. Moreover, women who substituted one serving of red meat per day for one serving of nuts lowered their risk of developing coronary heart disease by 30 percent, and substituting fish for red meat lowered their risk by 24 percent.

Older studies, too, communicate the inherent dangers of following a typical Western or American diet. During World War II, there was a marked reduction in the incidence of heart attacks in

CAUTION

Watch out for trans fat in milk and beef. A recent Norwegian study presented at the European Society of Cardiology's EuroPRevent meeting in Geneva revealed that small amounts of naturally occurring (ruminant) trans fats in milk and beef boost cardiac risk more than expected. The study of more than 71,000 people followed for twenty-five years showed that men with the highest consumption of ruminant trans fats were 41 percent more likely to die from coronary heart disease, and women with the highest ruminant trans fat intake were twice as likely to die from coronary heart disease.

Europe. Researchers have linked this finding to the marked decrease in red meat and dairy consumption during this time. When the war ended and red meat and dairy consumption returned, so did the heart attacks.

Research has also shown that following the toxic American diet leads to atherosclerotic coronary artery disease at a young age. The majority of the eighteen- to twenty-year-old soldiers killed in Vietnam and Korea already had established atherosclerotic plaques in their coronary arteries at the time of autopsy.

Other Meat Dangers

The trouble with meat is that it's not just the saturated fats and omega-6 fats that are harmful. Depending on what kinds of meats you like to eat, and how you cook them, you could be putting yourself at even greater risk.

Well-Done Is Not Done Well

Eating well-done meat has been found to increase the risk of certain cancers. Meats cooked at high temperatures generate chemicals called *heterocyclic amines* (HCAs). These HCAs are known to cause various cancers, including lung, bladder, colorectal, stomach, pancreatic, and others.

In one twelve-year study from the prestigious University of Texas MD Anderson Cancer Center, individuals who ate the most red meat were 1.5 times more likely to develop bladder cancer than those who ate the least red meat. Strikingly, the degree to which the meats were cooked also increased one's risk. Individuals who favored well-done meats were twice as likely to develop bladder cancer than meat-eaters who ate their cuts rare. Similar red meat eating patterns are also linked to lung cancer.

Processed Is Problematic (and Prohibited)

If you want to get serious about your cardiac makeover, there is one absolute rule: you *must* avoid processed meats. What I mean by *processed* is any meat that has been altered from its natural state for the sake of preserving its shelf life. Many researchers define processed meat as meat that is preserved by smoking, curing, or salting, or that includes the addition of chemical preservatives.

> Processed meats include:
> - Bacon
> - Deli or lunch meats
> - Hot dogs
> - Salami
> - Sausage

Want more proof? In 2010, the Harvard School of Public Health analyzed twenty studies covering a total of more than 1.2 million people from ten countries—possibly the largest study of its kind ever done. Researchers found that eating just one serving of processed meat per day was associated with a 42 percent higher risk of heart disease and 19 percent higher risk of developing diabetes.

The researchers noted in their article, published in *Circulation*, that the processed meats had, on average, four times more sodium and 50 percent more nitrate preservatives than unprocessed meats.

EASTERN DIETS COMPARED

A landmark study conducted by scientist T. Colin Campbell was one of the first to shine the spotlight on the toxicity of the typical meat-laden Western diet. He looked at mortality data on fifty diseases from more than 130 villages in rural mainland China. The results formed the basis for a book titled *The China Study*.

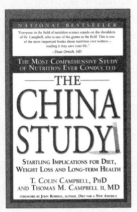

What he and his colleagues found was quite interesting. Chinese villagers consumed almost half the fat, 10 percent of the meat, and three times more fiber than Americans. When looking at cardiovascular parameters, the mean cholesterol count for the Chinese villagers was 127, compared to 203 for the U.S. population aged twenty to seventy-four. And death from coronary artery disease was almost seventeen times greater for American men and almost six times greater for American women compared to the respective populations of villagers.

Meat in Moderation

Based on my own experience and the overwhelming data showing the serious dangers of eating too much red meat, I tell my patients that if they must eat red meat, they should choose lean cuts, avoid cured or processed meats (bacon, deli meat, hot dogs, etc.)

Heart Attack Proof recommendations for red meat:

- Avoid regular red meat consumption (limit intake to 4 ounces two to four times a month)
- Avoid processed meat entirely
- Consume fish (omega-3 rich) and poultry (skinless chicken or turkey) several times per week

altogether, and eat small portions (no bigger than a deck of playing cards) no more than once a week.

If you want to be good to your heart, see lasting results from your cardiac makeover, and protect yourself from other diseases such as cancer, avoiding red meat consumption is one of the most important lifestyle changes you can make. The traditional Mediterranean diet is associated with infrequent red meat consumption (once or twice a month), and those who follow this diet have a fraction of the heart disease and cancer compared to the typical Western or American diet.

Dairy

One of our most prevalent American myths is that drinking whole milk every day is good for you. Besides increasing cholesterol due to its saturated fat content, whole milk has been a major contributor to the obesity epidemic in America. Did you know that three eight-ounce glasses of whole milk contains four-hundred-fifty calories and fifteen grams of saturated fat?

Regular milk consumption may increase the risk of:

- Diabetes
- GI disturbances (due to lactose intolerance)
- Heart disease
- Multiple sclerosis
- Ovarian cancer
- Prostate cancer

In addition, the hormones given to cows to increase their milk production, as well as the antibiotics they receive to prevent infection, are passed on to us through their milk—both have been found in the blood samples of milk drinkers.

If you consume cow's milk, switch from whole to fat-free or skim. Likewise, choose low-fat or fat-free cheese and yogurt.

Many milk alternatives are now available, including soy and almond milk. However, recent research has cautioned that, because soy milk contains phytoestrogens, it may not be suitable for women with a family history of breast cancer.

I recommend almond milk. Almonds are rich in nutrients, and almond milk has no cholesterol, saturated fat, or trans fat. In addition, almond milk is great for those who are lactose intolerant. Best of all, it's low-calorie and delicious!

The Mediterranean Diet:
The Optimal Diet for Heart Health

In contrast to the toxic American diet, the Mediterranean diet is very low in saturated fat and contains no trans fat. Despite the name, there is nothing exotic about it. All of the foods found in a traditional Mediterranean diet are in your supermarket or grocery store.

The diet consists of fruits, vegetables, olive oil, whole grains, legumes, nuts, fish, poultry, and red wine (in moderation), and is plentiful in the vitamins, fiber, and antioxidants required for good health. Red meat is eaten infrequently, and refined sugar and processed foods are avoided. As previously noted, this diet includes many foods that have been shown to reduce inflammation, whereas the foods in the traditional American diet *promote* inflammation. Decreasing inflammation lowers the risk of heart disease, cancer, diabetes, and a host of other diseases that are linked to chronic low-grade inflammation.

The result is that those who enjoy this type of diet seem to be essentially protected from heart disease. In addition, clinical studies have demonstrated that switching from a highly processed Western or American diet to a traditional Mediterranean diet results in sustained weight loss and improvements in overall health. Finally, this diet lowers the risk of metabolic syndrome, diabetes, hypertension, Alzheimer's disease, cancer, and a number of other diseases.

Best of all, a Mediterranean diet is delicious and can be enjoyed by the entire family.

The Mediterranean Diet (and Lifestyle) Pyramid

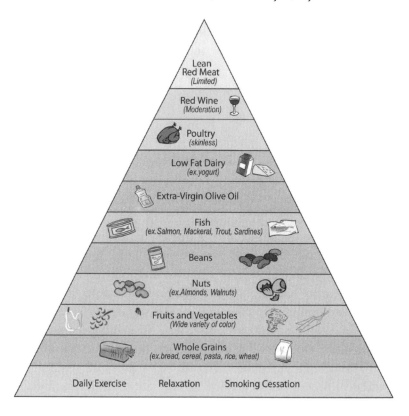

A Mediterranean diet can also be a great tool for weight loss. People who live in the Mediterranean region and follow a traditional Mediterranean diet and lifestyle are much leaner than their American counterparts who consume a typical highly processed Western diet.

This diet and the wonderful foods it offers promote weight loss in a number of ways:

- *It's high in fiber.* The consumption of food with high fiber content (fruits, vegetables, beans, nuts, and whole grains) leads to feelings of satiety, or being full and satisfied, so you consume fewer calories.

- *It promotes omega-3 thermogenesis.* The consumption of omega-3 fats has been shown to help achieve weight loss through a process known as thermogenesis, or heat release following the metabolism of fat.
- *It contains less sugar.* The Mediterranean diet contains complex instead of simple carbohydrates, and refined sugar is avoided. Only 3 percent of a traditional Mediterranean diet contains added sugar, compared to 25 percent of most American diets.

THE MIAMI MEDITERRANEAN DIET

Are you wondering, "How am I going to find additional information regarding the Mediterranean diet and how am I going to learn how to prepare the recipes?" Relax! To get you started, I've included a 7-Day Meal Plan complete with recipes in Appendix C. This meal plan is taken, in part, from my previous book, *The Miami Mediterranean Diet*, which offers hundreds of delicious recipes that are easy to prepare and will satisfy the entire family, 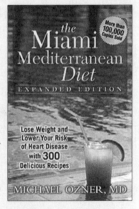 and it includes a wide variety of meals, from breakfast, lunch, and dinner to heart-healthy snacks and desserts. Join the thousands of others who have utilized *The Miami Mediterranean Diet* to achieve optimal health and weight control!

THE SKINNY ON SWEETENERS

Until recently, options for calorie-free sweeteners had all been chemical: Equal, Sweet'N Low, and Splenda are all chemical derivatives of sugar, but are not natural.

The good news is that natural zero-calorie sweeteners are now being made from the stevia plant. The stevia plant's leaves, from which the sweeteners are made, are known to be thirty times sweeter than table sugar. Brands like Truvia, Pure Via, and others can now be found at most major grocery stores. A little goes a long way, so try some in your tea or coffee. You can even use it for baking!

Building Your New Diet: A Mediterranean Mix

In short, the Mediterranean diet and lifestyle provides a great foundation for healthy living that promotes weight loss and maintenance. For all these reasons, it's the diet and lifestyle I have recommended to my patients for over twenty-five years.

Let's now take a closer look at the healthy and delicious foods of the Mediterranean diet.

Good Fats: Omega-3 Fatty Acids

Omega-3 fat is an important component of the Mediterranean diet because it is something the average American doesn't consume enough of. It has been suggested that up to 90 percent of Americans are deficient in omega-3 fatty acids.

Why should this matter? Whereas omega-6 fat (found in vegetable oil and much of today's red meat) is pro-inflammatory, omega-3 fat (found in walnuts, flaxseed oil, and fish) is anti-inflammatory. The omega-6/omega-3 ratio in our diet should be 2/1 to maintain optimal health; however, due to a dietary decrease in omega-3 intake and increase in omega-6 intake, for many of us that ratio is somewhere between 10/1 and 20/1. The Mediterranean diet naturally resets this ratio to healthy levels by providing your body with ample amounts of omega-3 fat.

Omega-3 deficiency can lead to an increase in:
- Acne
- Allergies
- Arthritis
- Asthma
- Cancer
- Depression
- Diabetes
- Heart disease
- Heart rhythm disorders
- Hypertension
- Inflammatory bowel disease
- Sudden cardiac death

Olive Oil

Olive oil, which is made by crushing and then pressing olives, is the "soul" of the Mediterranean diet and provides the taste and flavor of many Mediterranean dishes. It is rich in monounsaturated fat and an excellent substitute for butter or margarine.

Olive oil also has a favorable impact on cholesterol. Besides decreasing total cholesterol, it lowers (bad) LDL cholesterol without lowering (good) HDL cholesterol, which improves the total-cholesterol-to-HDL-cholesterol ratio. Olive oil has also been shown to have beneficial anti-inflammatory, antioxidant, and anti-thrombotic properties.

Olive oil also helps with weight loss. A study in Boston revealed that a diet that included olive oil and nuts resulted in sustained weight loss over eighteen months compared to a low-fat diet. People also stayed on the diet longer because they did not feel deprived.

One word of caution despite these favorable effects: olive oil is highly caloric (100 calories per tablespoon) and contains mainly monounsaturated fat. A study reported by Dr. Lawrence Rudel of Wake Forest University demonstrated that a regular large intake of monounsaturated fat can lead to the development of atherosclerosis

COOKING AT HIGH HEAT? TRY CANOLA OIL

Canola oil has a high smoke point, which means it can be used for cooking at high temperatures, like stir-frying. In addition, it is a good source of alpha-linolenic acid, an omega-3 fat.

in non-human primates. As noted earlier in this chapter: be sure to only use olive oil in moderation—drizzle, don't pour!

Vinegar

Vinegar has long been a staple of the Mediterranean diet. It is frequently used with olive oil on salads and vegetables, and for a good reason: like olive oil, vinegar leads to satiety.

In addition, vinegar helps manage blood sugar and insulin levels: it helps reduce blood glucose by delaying food from leaving the stomach, which slows the absorption of carbohydrates. Researchers reported in the *European Journal of Clinical Nutrition* that when subjects were served vinegar with white bread, their blood sugar and insulin levels were lower than those of subjects who consumed white bread without vinegar.

Fresh Fruits and Vegetables

Go to any supermarket in the Mediterranean basin and you will find a bountiful supply of fresh, native fruits and vegetables. Fruits and vegetables contain an abundance of vitamins, minerals, fiber, and complex carbohydrates that lower the risk of heart disease and cancer. They also contain phytonutrients, concentrated in the skins, which help fight disease and improve health.

In a large European study, published in the *European Heart Journal* and involving 313,074 men and women from eight European countries who were followed for more than eight years, those who ate at least eight servings of fruits and vegetables per day had a 22 percent lower risk of dying from coronary heart disease than those who ate fewer than three servings a day. Adding just one additional fruit or vegetable serving per day decreased risk by 4 percent.

Whole Grains

Whole grains are non-processed grains that retain fiber, nutrients, and a heartier, nuttier texture than their refined counterparts. Grains in the Mediterranean basin are not processed (or are only minimally processed) and therefore retain their nutrients. A whole grain kernel consists of an outer layer, the bran (fiber); a middle layer (complex carbohydrates and protein); and an inner layer (vitamins, minerals, and proteins). The process of refining destroys the outer and inner layer of the grain, resulting in a stripped version that is devoid of the healthy fiber and protective vitamins and phytochemicals. Because they retain more fiber, vitamins, and phytochemicals, whole grains have been shown to decrease the risk of heart disease and diabetes.

Some of my favorite heart-healthy fruits and vegetables:

- Artichoke
- Zucchini
- Eggplant
- Spinach
- Red peppers
- Mushrooms
- Garlic
- Olives
- Chickpeas
- Orange
- Apples
- Grapes
- Pomegranate

Common whole grains include:

- Wheat
- Buckwheat
- Oats
- Brown Rice
- Quinoa
- Rye
- Amaranth
- Spelt
- Millet
- Maize

Common whole grain products include:

- Whole wheat bread
- Whole wheat pasta
- Whole wheat flour
- Rolled oats

A recent study conducted by Harvard's School of Public Health found that eating five or more servings of white rice per week is associated with an increased risk of type-2 diabetes. But if the white rice is changed to brown rice, the risk is lowered. When the white rice was replaced with other whole grains such as whole wheat and barley, the risk decreased even further.

Nuts and Beans

Nuts are an excellent source of good fats and protein and are frequently consumed as part of a Mediterranean diet. For example, almonds are rich in fiber, and walnuts contain heart-healthy omega-3 fat. Several clinical trials have demonstrated that consuming nuts in moderation on a regular basis leads to lower cholesterol, a decreased risk of coronary heart disease, and a significant reduction in the risk of heart attack. I recommend a handful of natural raw almonds or walnuts every day as a satisfying and nutritious midday snack.

Beans and legumes are another good source of protein and fiber. They too have been shown to lower the risk of heart disease, cancer, and diabetes when consumed regularly.

THE ADVENTIST HEALTH STUDY

In the Adventist Health Study, an investigation of more than 31,000 Seventh-Day Adventists, subjects who consumed nuts (specifically almonds) frequently—more than four times per week—experienced substantially fewer fatal and non-fatal heart attacks than those who consumed nuts less than once per week. Their relative risk of a heart attack was reduced by 50 percent!

FISH CONSUMPTION AND CARDIOVASCULAR HEALTH

In the US Physicians Health Study, weekly fish consumption was associated with a 50 percent lower risk of sudden cardiac death. In addition, a study by researchers from the Harvard School of Public Health, published in the *Journal of the American Medical Association* in 2006, concluded that the cardiovascular and overall health benefits of weekly fish consumption greatly outweigh the risks.

Fish

What would a Mediterranean diet be without fish? The Mediterranean Sea offers a variety of omega-3-rich seafood that is exceptionally healthy. When looking for the optimal health benefits, oily, cold-water fish are your best bets, as they have the highest levels of omega-3 fat. In particular, salmon is an excellent choice, as well as albacore tuna, herring, sardines, shad, trout, flounder (or sole), and pollock.

A note of caution, however: Avoid eating swordfish, tilefish, shark, and mackerel, as these tend to have very high mercury levels. (See Appendix B for a list of fish and other seafood and their omega-3 and mercury levels.) It is particularly important that women who are pregnant or nursing and young children avoid fish with high mercury levels. Always discuss nutritional recommendations, including fish consumption, with your healthcare provider.

Alcohol

By now I've covered the pros and cons of red meat, dairy, fruits and vegetables, fish, olive oil and vinegar, and more. So now I offer up a toast to the good life with a glass of red wine, or even your favorite evening alcoholic beverage. Cultures with the longest longevity—including those living in the Mediterranean—all have been known to drink small amounts of alcohol every day. Indeed, daily consumption of alcohol in moderation has been shown to decrease the risk of heart attack up to 45 percent!

Countless studies have shown the cardiovascular benefits of drinking a glass of red wine with dinner. Part of that reason may be that red wine raises (good) HDL cholesterol, decreases clotting, lowers inflammation, and reduces oxidation of (bad) LDL cholesterol. In addition, red wine also contains resveratrol, a powerful antioxidant.

Furthermore, new data shows that other types of alcohol, including beer and spirits, also provide protection against heart disease. In an INTER-HEART study involving 27,000 people from fifty-two countries, light to moderate drinking reduced the incidence of heart attack in men and women in all age groups, regardless of alcohol type. Moderate alcohol consumption also decreased the risk of ischemic stroke and type-2 diabetes.

An evening drink has also been shown to be beneficial in those with cardiovascular risk factors, such as hypertension. In one study that tracked 11,711 men with hypertension over sixteen years, one drink per day reduced the risk of a heart attack by about 30 percent. However, the study also showed that moderation was key: those who had more than two drinks daily showed increases in blood pressure. That's right—alcohol, including red wine, only has cardiovascular benefits when consumed in moderation: one glass per day for women and two glasses per day for men. (One glass means 5 oz of wine, 12 oz of beer, or 1.5 oz of spirits.) Men and women who exceed moderation raise their risk of heart disease, liver disease, and cancer.

One other word of caution: Women who consume alcohol have been shown to increase their risk of breast cancer. There is, however, scientific evidence that adequate consumption of vitamin B9

TOAST TO YOUR HEART: HEART-HEALTHY DRINKING

1. Drink just before or with your evening meal.
2. Consume no more than one drink for a woman, or two drinks for a man in a twenty-four-hour period.
3. One drink equals 12 oz of beer, 5 oz of wine, or 1.5 oz of spirits.

(folate or folic acid) may reduce or eliminate that risk. The evidence comes from a study of over 17,000 Australian women aged forty to sixty-nine over a period of about ten years. Women who regularly consumed alcohol and took 200 micrograms of vitamin B9 every day had a lower risk of breast cancer than women who abstained from alcohol. Foods rich in folate include citrus fruits, dark green leafy vegetables, dried beans, and peas. Most daily multiple vitamins also contain vitamin B9.

Abuse of alcohol can lead to:

- Addiction
- Auto and other accidents
- Cirrhosis of the liver
- Depression
- Heart rhythm disturbances
- Increased risk of certain cancers
- Insomnia
- Memory Loss

As a preventive cardiologist, I do not encourage my patients who don't drink alcohol to start drinking in order to reduce their risk of a heart attack; there are better ways to lower risk without the potential adverse effects of alcohol. I do, however, advise my patients who already consume alcohol to do so in moderation.

Grape Juice—A Non-Alcoholic Alternative to Red Wine

For those of you who don't wish to drink red wine or other forms of alcohol but still want the cardiovascular benefits, don't dismay—grape juice may be your answer. Research has shown that

Concord grape juice:

- Decreases blood pressure
- Decreases inflammation
- Decreases LDL oxidation
- Decreases oxidative stress
- Decreases platelet aggregation
- Improves cholesterol
- Improves endothelial function
- Increases nitrous oxide production

Concord grape juice can provide beneficial cardiovascular effects similar to red wine.

Dr. Joseph Vita and colleagues demonstrated that Concord grape juice had a beneficial effect on blood pressure. It has also been shown to increase nitric oxide production in the endothelial cells that line the arteries producing a vasodilating effect. This promotes arterial relaxation and flexibility, which has a beneficial impact on blood pressure and arterial function.

Other beneficial effects of Concord grape juice consumption:

- *It improves cognitive function.* A study from the University of Cincinnati College of Medicine to determine whether Concord grape juice would be beneficial in patients with age-related cognitive decline demonstrated improvement in short-term retention and spatial memory. Research conducted at Mt. Sinai School of Medicine found that polyphenols from Concord grape juice decreased the generation and accumulation of beta-amyloid peptides in experimental models of Alzheimer's disease. Beta-amyloid peptides are known to accumulate in the brain in patients with Alzheimer's disease and lead to plaque formation.
- *It aids in weight control.* A twelve-week study by Hollis and colleagues demonstrated that Concord grape juice not only did not cause significant weight gain, but actually reduced waist circumference.
- *It's anti-thrombotic.* Clinical studies have shown that Concord grape juice decreases blood clotting.

Tea

Don't let your love affair with coffee blind you to the benefits of tea, a beverage frequently consumed in Mediterranean countries. Both coffee and tea contain antioxidants and chemicals that have been found to reduce the risk of diabetes, gallstones, and kidney stones. But only tea contains substances that help reduce the risk of heart disease and cancer.

One question I am often asked is whether the kind of tea matters. The answer is yes. All teas come from the *camellia sinensis* plant, and the way the leaves are processed determines the tea's type and color. Green tea is made from young leaves that are immediately steamed, rolled, and dried. Black tea comes from leaves that are exposed to oxygen for two to four hours. White tea is the least processed and lowest in caffeine. Green tea is usually lauded as the healthiest because its processing provides more antioxidant power, however black and white tea also have significant health benefits.

Researchers at the University of California in Los Angeles conducted a meta-analysis of several studies comparing stroke protection in green tea and black tea drinkers. The results suggested that daily consumption of either green or black tea (three cups per day) could help prevent ischemic stroke.

Chinese researchers recently analyzed eighteen tea studies published in the *American Journal of Clinical Nutrition* and determined that while black tea is definitely healthy, green tea is still best if you want to decrease your risk of dying from heart disease. In their analysis, an increase of green tea consumption of one cup per day was associated with a 10 percent decrease in the risk of developing coronary artery disease.

To release tea's strongest health benefits, brew it yourself, using either the leaves or a tea bag, and let it steep in the cup for three to five minutes. Keep in mind that while herbal teas may be more flavorful, pure tea packs a stronger antioxidant punch.

Cinnamon

A variety of spices are used in the Mediterranean diet, including cinnamon, which is made from the bark of the cinnamon tree and contains three types of essential oils that provide it with health-boosting properties. These oils act as an anti-coagulant, preventing blood from forming dangerous clots; they have anti-inflammatory properties; and they enhance the ability of diabetics to metabolize sugar.

In fact, less than half a teaspoon a day of cinnamon can lower glucose levels and improve cholesterol balance in people at high risk for diabetes and coronary heart disease. There's even some research indicating that just the smell of cinnamon can help improve brain activity.

Specific Health Benefits
of a Traditional Mediterranean Diet

This week is about building a new dietary and nutritional foundation for you to lose weight (or to maintain your current weight) while reaping the wealth of health benefits a Mediterranean-style diet has to offer.

In fact, researchers from Italy recently looked at all the studies through June 2010 that assessed the benefits of the Mediterranean diet and published them in the *American Journal of Clinical Nutrition*. They found that the Mediterranean diet was associated with a statistically significant reduction of overall mortality, as well as cardiovascular and cancer mortality.

Improved Cardiovascular Health

We've already mentioned some of the cardio-protective effects of the Mediterranean diet. Some of the landmark studies confirming the benefits include:

The Lyon Diet Heart Study

This study compared a Mediterranean diet to a control diet (resembling the American Heart Association's Step 1 diet). The control diet is still considered healthy, since it restricted total fat to no more than 30 percent of total calories, saturated fat to no more than 10 percent of total calories, and cholesterol to less than 300 mg/day. However, the Mediterranean diet was healthier. It had more whole grain bread, more vegetables, and more fish, as well as less beef, lamb, and pork (which were replaced with poultry). It included at least one serving of fruit every day, and butter and cream were replaced with a spread high in omega-3 fat.

> The Mediterranean diet helps prevent:
>
> - Cardiovascular disease
> - Hypertension
> - Alzheimer's disease
> - Allergies
> - Asthma
> - Autoimmune diseases
> - Cancer
> - Diabetes
> - Depression and anxiety
> - Inflammatory bowel disease
> - Metabolic Syndrome
> - Neurodegenerative diseases

The Mediterranean diet proved far superior to the control diet—it was associated with a 70 percent decrease in the risk of death and 73 percent decrease in the risk of recurrent cardiac events such as heart attack or sudden cardiac death.

The Singh Indo-Mediterranean Diet Study

This study placed 499 patients who were at risk for coronary heart disease on a Mediterranean diet. Results showed that the diet reduced cholesterol and also significantly reduced heart attacks and sudden cardiac death.

The NIH-AARP Diet and Health Study

This study looked at more than 350,000 men and women in the United States to evaluate the impact of a Mediterranean diet on their health. The findings, published in the 2007 *Archives of Internal Medicine*, demonstrated that a Mediterranean diet not only lowered the risk of heart attacks, but also significantly reduced the death rate from a variety of diseases, including cardiovascular disease and cancer. These results provide strong evidence for a beneficial effect of the Mediterranean diet on the risk of death from all causes.

Protection Against Cancer

The beauty of the traditional Mediterranean diet is that it is synergistic in how it protects the body. This means that not only is each component nutritious in and of itself, but when they are combined, they become even more effective. This may help explain why this diet has shown significant protection against certain types of cancer.

Recent research from Harvard University, published July 2010 in the *American Journal of Clinical Nutrition*, showed that 14,800 Greek women who followed a traditional Mediterranean diet most closely were 22 percent less likely to develop breast cancer than those who ate less traditional diets. These results echo other research showing protection against colon, stomach, and prostate cancer by following the Mediterranean diet.

Protection Against Alzheimer's Disease

Dr. Nikolaos Scarmeas and colleagues from Columbia University Medical Center in New York demonstrated in 2006 that a Mediterranean diet reduced the risk of developing Alzheimer's disease by 68 percent. Recent updates to this study confirm the original results and also show that the Mediterranean diet may reduce the risk of mild cognitive impairment.

A third, related study by Scarmeas looking at diet, exercise, and Alzheimer's risk in elderly French participants showed that the greater the adherence to a Mediterranean diet and regular exercise, the lower the risk for developing Alzheimer's disease.

Reduced Depression Rates

The benefits of the Mediterranean diet go beyond reduced rates of heart disease, helping prevent cancer, and offering protection against Alzheimer's disease. The lifetime incidence of depression in Mediterranean countries is lower than in northern European countries, according to research published in *Archives of General Psychiatry* by Spanish scientists. In approximately 10,000 healthy Spanish people followed for six years, those who adhered to a Mediterranean diet saw a 30 percent reduction in the risk of becoming depressed compared to those who did not follow a Mediterranean-style diet.

Assignment #1: Commit to a Mediterranean Diet

The evidence is clear: Following a Mediterranean diet is one of the very best things you can do for your cardiovascular health. This week, I want you to commit to doing so.

The Mediterranean diet is not difficult to adhere to—its colorful, fresh, and wholesome food is easy to find, easy to prepare, and, most importantly, delicious! To get you started is the 7-Day Meal Plan in Appendix C that will teach you to prepare heart-healthy meals—from breakfast to lunch and dinner, as well as snacks between meals. Hundreds of additional recipes are available in *The Miami Mediterranean Diet.*

And don't worry, I'm not asking you to give up going out to eat. Appendix D is a "survival guide" to help you consume heart-healthy fare even when you're out at your favorite restaurant. Bon Appetit!

Assignment #2: Face the Scales

This week it's important for you to take an honest look at your weight and your BMI, and if you need to lose weight, make a commitment to do so. Losing weight is really just a matter of calories taken in versus calories burned. Generally, 3,500 calories burned equals one pound of weight lost. This is why it is so important to stay active, and to choose your calories carefully. Consuming highly processed, calorie-dense, and nutrient-depleted food is doing your body a big disservice. If you wouldn't put diesel fuel in your gasoline-powered car, why would you put highly processed food in your body? The wrong fuel in your car results in a mechanical breakdown of your vehicle and costly repairs. The wrong food in your body leads to disease and even costlier treatment.

Be Realistic and Succeed!

When trying to lose weight, be realistic—losing a large amount of weight in a short time is unhealthy and cannot be sustained. Try to lose one to two pounds per week. This may sound very modest, but over the course of a year that can lead to fifty to one hundred

RAPID WEIGHT LOSS

Be smart—don't try to lose a large amount of weight in a short period of time. Extreme short-term weight loss is usually associated with fluid and electrolyte loss, which leads to dehydration. This is not healthy and can lead to serious side effects like heart rhythm disturbances and kidney malfunction.

pounds of weight loss! Achieving a healthy weight is about committing to a lifestyle change—eating the right foods and getting regular exercise.

To shed one pound means you must burn (or eliminate) an extra 3,500 calories per week, or 500 calories per day. Start with the easy stuff: one soda contains 150 calories, so a perfect way to reduce 500 calories per day would be to cut out two sodas and walk for approximately thirty to forty-five minutes.

The Bathroom Scale

I doubt that you ever ran out of gas while driving your car because you forgot to look at the fuel gauge. Yet most of us forget to look at the "fuel gauge" for our bodies—the bathroom scale. Weigh yourself daily and strive for one to two pounds of weight loss per week. If you aren't able to achieve this goal, you have three choices:

- Eat less.
- Exercise more.
- Eat less and exercise more.

Eating less does not mean that you walk around hungry. Remember, staples of the Mediterranean diet include fruits, vegetables, beans, and nuts—foods that, while low in calories, are rich in fiber that leads to satiety.

Don't get discouraged if you notice mild fluctuation in your weight from week to week, as factors such as fluid retention (especially in women) can cause transient weight gain. Remember, the important thing is to gradually achieve your ideal body weight over time by forming new habits that will keep the weight off.

WEEK 4

Putting It Into Practice

You've stopped smoking, seen your doctor and dentist, begun a regular exercise program, and learned how to reduce stress and relax. You've also started making changes to what you eat, and this week you'll be committing to a Mediterranean diet, which will not only improve your health, but will also help you achieve your ideal body weight.

This week, you should:

☐ Reduce your (lean) red meat consumption to once a week—or less.

☐ Begin to avoid processed meat entirely.

☐ Enjoy a glass of red wine with dinner.

☐ Use olive oil instead of butter or margarine (but drizzle, don't pour!).

☐ Use whole grain bread in place of highly processed, refined white bead.

☐ Try at least two recipes from the Heart Healthy 7-Day Meal Plan in Appendix C.

☐ Assess your weight and BMI, and begin your path toward ideal body weight.

Know Your Numbers

We've never had a heart attack in Framingham in thirty-five years in anyone who had a cholesterol level under 150 ... Three-quarters of the people who live on the face of the Earth never have a heart attack. They live in Asia, Africa and South America, and their cholesterols are all around 150.

—Dr. William Castelli,
Medical Director, Framingham Cardiovascular Institute

I N WEEK 1, you set up an appointment with your doctor for a routine physical as well as comprehensive blood tests. This week, I will help you learn what each of the values on your test results means, so that you can take better control of your health and play an active role in maintaining your cardiovascular well-being. Achieving optimal blood chemistry is essential to becoming Heart Attack Proof.

Why It's Important to Get Cardiovascular Blood Tests

The best way to detect metabolic abnormalities, like elevated (bad) LDL cholesterol particles or increased vascular inflammation (which may be present even if you feel well) is through a blood test. Detecting metabolic disorders is particularly important for uncovering hidden risk for heart attack, stroke, and vascular disease, thereby allowing physicians to individualize treatment programs that will lower patients' risk of disability and death from cardiovascular disease. Simply using a standard lipid or cholesterol profile (total cholesterol, [bad] LDL cholesterol, [good] HDL cholesterol, and triglycerides) uncovers 40 percent of heart attack risk, whereas an expanded cardiovascular risk profile, with tests such as LDL particle number and hs-CRP, can uncover 90 percent of heart attack risk. Performing regular blood tests is also essential for effectively monitoring already diagnosed conditions and ensuring that medical treatment and lifestyle changes are working.

The cost of comprehensive blood tests has decreased significantly over the past several years. And compared to the cost of treating heart attack, stroke, or peripheral vascular disease—that is, compared to the potential cost of not knowing what's going on in your body and only being able to treat these conditions once they strike—it's a steal!

The best time to have a comprehensive laboratory evaluation is when you are feeling well. If you wait until a heart attack (or stroke) strikes, you've waited too long. One-third of men and women do not survive their first heart attack, and those who do have to undergo expensive interventional procedures and lengthy hospital stays that can cost between $50,000 and $100,000. Long-term care can be very expensive, and the loss of your future earning potential can be significant. Prevention of atherosclerosis and heart attack or stroke is one of the most cost-effective strategies available—not to mention the nonfinancial benefits of staying healthy and productive and enjoying life.

SUDDEN DEATH

The initial presentation of coronary artery disease in up to one-third of patients is sudden death.

Half of all heart attack patients have a normal (bad) LDL cholesterol.

It is reasonable to check with your insurance carrier to see what tests are covered and what your out-of-pocket cost will be. Just remember: an investment in your health is one of the best investments you can make!

Let's take a look at the blood test results for one of my patients, Max, so you can see exactly how important it is to have these tests done and understand the results.

Patient Profile: Max

Max was not the type of person you would expect to have a heart attack at age thirty-six—but he did. Married and the father of two daughters, Max always considered himself to be healthy. He was active in his real estate law practice, and he played tennis or golf on most weekends.

I first met Max in the emergency room when asked to do an emergency consult at the time of his heart attack. He told me that he had never experienced chest pain in the past and he always had an annual checkup with his family doctor. He went on to tell me that his cholesterol levels were always low and that he had passed a stress test a year ago. Max's father had had a mild heart attack at the age of sixty-nine; otherwise his family history was unremarkable.

Max was overweight but not obese, and his BMI was 28. His waist circumference was forty-two inches, and he had mild hypertension. His blood pressure was 145/92.

When I reviewed Max's prior lab work it became clear that he was not an unfortunate soul who just happened to have an unexpected heart attack. Rather, he was like millions of Americans: a "ticking time bomb" just waiting to have a cardiovascular catastrophe. How did I know this? Simply by looking at his lab values from six months prior:

Total cholesterol: 166
LDL cholesterol: 90
HDL cholesterol: 36
Triglycerides: 200
Fasting blood sugar: 112

It was clear that Max had metabolic syndrome, a condition that put him at high risk for a future cardiac event. In fact, Max hit the jackpot—he had *all five* features of metabolic syndrome.

When I told Max that, he was astonished. "I always thought I was at low risk for a heart attack, since my cholesterol was always less than 200 and my blood sugar was always normal or just mildly elevated," he said. I explained to Max that he was walking around with insulin resistance and the associated lipid abnormalities of high triglycerides and low (good) HDL cholesterol. I also hypothesized that when we tested his blood, we would find that he had an excessive amount of small dense LDL particles, which are almost always associated with insulin resistance and metabolic syndrome.

I was correct. When I measured Max's LDL particle number, it was markedly elevated: 2600. So despite having an annual physical exam and blood analysis and being told that his cholesterol was low, he had thousands of small (LDL) cholesterol particles that were causing atherosclerotic plaques in his coronary artery walls. Unfortunately, one of those plaques had suddenly ruptured, leading to Max's heart attack.

WHAT IS METABOLIC SYNDROME?

Metabolic Syndrome is a cluster of metabolic abnormalities—impaired fasting glucose, low (good) HDL cholesterol, and elevated triglycerides—along with abdominal obesity and an increased blood pressure, all conditions that lead to premature heart attack, stroke, and vascular disease. Presently one in four Americans has metabolic syndrome—and that number is increasing, both here and around the world, due to rising obesity rates and sedentary lifestyles.

Metabolic syndrome means you have at least three of the following five conditions:

- Abdominal obesity (waist circumference > 40 inches for men or > 35 inches for women)
- High levels of triglycerides (> 150 mg/dl)
- Low levels of (good) HDL cholesterol (< 40 mg/dl for men or < 50 mg/dl for women)
- Elevated blood pressure (> 130/85 mm/hg)
- Elevated fasting glucose (> 100 mg/dl)

The optimal approach for the treatment, prevention, and reversal of metabolic syndrome is a healthy lifestyle with regular exercise and a heart-healthy (Mediterranean) diet.

Before Max left the hospital, I ordered a comprehensive blood test to assess his risk for a future heart attack. When he returned for the results, he was amazed. He had so many abnormal metabolic parameters, he wondered why he did not have a heart attack years ago. The numbers told the story:

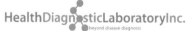

Laboratory Test	Notes	High Risk	Intermediate Risk	Optimal	High Risk Range	Intermediate Risk Range	Optimal Range	Previous Results
Lipids								
Total Cholesterol (mg/dL)				156	≥ 240	200 - 239	< 200	
LDL-C Direct (mg/dL)				73	≥ 130 CHD & CHD risk eq. > 100	100 - 129 CHD & CHD risk eq. 70 - 100	< 100 CHD & CHD risk eq. < 70	
HDL-C (mg/dL)		35			< 40		≥ 40	
Triglycerides (mg/dL)			175		≥ 200	150 - 199	< 150	
Non-HDL-C (mg/dL) (calculated)				121	≥ 160	130 - 159	< 130	
Lipoprotein Particles and Apolipoproteins								
Apo B (mg/dL)		125			≥ 80	60 - 79	< 60	
LDL-P (nmol/L)		2600			≥ 1300	1000 - 1299	< 1000	
sdLDL (mg/dL)*		38			≥ 31	21 - 30	≤ 20	
Apo A-I (mg/dL)		92			< 114	114 - 131	≥ 132	
HDL-P (µmol/L)		25.0			< 28.0	28.0 - 34.0	≥ 35.0	
HDL2 (mg/dL)*		8			≤ 8	9 - 11	≥ 12	
Apo B:Apo A-I Ratio (calculated)		1.36			≥ 0.81	0.61 - 0.81	≤ 0.6	
Lp(a) Mass (mg/dL)				22	≥ 30		< 30	
Lp(a) Cholesterol (mg/dL)					≥ 6	3 - 5	< 3	
Inflammation/ Oxidation								
Myeloperoxidase (pmol/L)		552			≥ 550	400 - 549	< 400	
Lp-PLA₂ (ng/mL)		285			> 235	200 - 235	< 200	
hs-CRP (mg/L)			2.8		≥ 3.0	1.0 - 2.9	< 1.0	
Fibrinogen (mg/dL)					≥ 465	391 - 464	≤ 390	
Myocardial Stress								
NT-proBNP (pg/mL)					≥ 450	125 - 449	< 125	
Platelets								
AspirinWorks® (urine) (pg/mg of creatinine)					> 1500		≤ 1500	

Lab Notes:

Provider Notes:

www.myhdl.com

Dr. Joseph P. McConnell | Laboratory Director | CLIA No. 49D1100708 | CAP No. 7224971 | NPI No. 1629209853

©2010 | 737 N. 5th Street Suite 103 | Richmond, Virginia 23219 | Phone: 804.343.2718 | Fax: 804.343.2704

HDL 20.0

To schedule time with a Personal Health Coach, please call 1-877-443-5227) or visit us online at www.myhdl.com

HealthDiagnosticLaboratoryInc.
beyond disease diagnosis

Laboratory Results

Patient

Name: Max Test	Phone #:	Patient ID #:
Fasting Status:	Gender:	Birthdate:	Age:
Height:	Weight:	BMI:	Prev. BMI:

Specimen

Collection Time:	Specimen ID:
Collection Date:	Report Type:
Received Date:	Report Date:

Provider

| Requesting Provider: |
| Client ID: |

Laboratory Test	Notes	High Risk	Intermediate Risk	Optimal	High Risk Range	Intermediate Risk Range	Optimal Range	Previous Results
Lipoprotein Genetics Apolipoprotein E Genotype*					Estimated Genotype Frequency: 2/2 (~1-2%), 2/3 (~15%), 2/4 (~1-2%), 3/3 (~55%), 3/4 (~25%), 4/4 (~1-2%)			
Platelet Genetics CYP2C19*2*3* POOR metabolizers with poor antiplatelet effect of Plavix.					*1/*1 = optimal, *1/*2 or *1/*3 = intermediate, *2/*2, *2/*3 or *3/*3 = poor			
CYP2C19*17* RAPID metabolizers at increased risk for bleeding on Plavix.					*1/*1 = optimal, *1/*17 = rapid, *17/*17 = ultra rapid			
Coagulation Genetics Factor V Leiden					**Optimal**=Non-carrier (Arg/Arg); **At Risk**=(Arg/Gln or Gln/Gln)			
Prothrombin Mutation					**Optimal**=Non-carrier (G/G); **At Risk**=(G/A or A/A)			
Metabolic Insulin (µU/mL)					≥ 12	10 - 11	3 - 9	
Free Fatty Acid (mmol/L)					> 0.7	0.6 - 0.7	≤ 0.59	
Glucose (mg/dL)			106		≤ 55 or > 125	56-69 or 100-125	70 - 99	
HbA1c (%)			6.2		≥ 6.5	5.7 - 6.4	≤ 5.6	
Estimated Average Glucose (mg/dL) (calculated)			131.2		≥ 139.9	116.9 - 139.8	≤ 116.8	
25-hydroxy-Vitamin D (ng/mL)		11			≤ 14	15 - 29	30 - 100	
TSH (µIU/mL)				2.43	< 0.27 or > 4.20		0.27 - 4.20	
Homocysteine (µmol/L)					> 13	11 - 13	≤ 10	
Renal Creatinine, serum (mg/dL)				1.2	> 1.2		0.7 - 1.2	

Lab Notes:

To schedule time with a Personal Health Coach, please call 1-877-4HDLABS (1-877-443-5227) or visit us online at www.myhdl.com

Dr. Joseph P. McCo___ll | Laboratory Director | CLIA No. 49D1100708 | CAP No. 7224971 | NPI No. 1629209853
©2010 | 737 N. 5th Street Suite 103 | Richmond, Virginia 23219 | Phone: 804.343.2718 | Fax: 804.343.2704

HDL 20.0

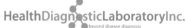

HealthDiagnosticLaboratoryInc.
beyond disease diagnosis

Laboratory Results

Patient

Name: Max Test
Phone #:
Patient ID #:

Fasting Status:
Gender:
Birthdate:
Age:

Height:
Weight:
BMI:
Prev. BMI:

Specimen

Collection Time:
Specimen ID:

Collection Date:
Report Type:

Received Date:
Report Date:

Provider

Requesting Provider:

Client ID:

Other Biomarkers	Result	Flag	Reference Interval
Albumin (g/dl)	4.3		3.5 - 5.2
ALP (U/L)	77		40 - 129
ALT / GPT (U/L)	38		Up to 41
AST / GOT (U/L)	37		Up to 40
BUN (mg/dl)	18		6 - 20
Calcium (mg/dL)	9.7		8.6 - 10.2
Cl- (mmol/L)	101		96 - 108
CO_2 (mmol/L)	27		22 - 29
K+ (mmol/L)	5.1		3.3 - 5.1
Na+ (mmol/L)	141		133 - 145
Total Bilirubin (mg/dL)	1.1		Up to 1.2
Total Protein (g/dL)	6.9		6.4 - 8.3
T4 (µg/dL)	4.9		4.5 - 11.7
T3 (ng/dL)	99		80 - 200

CBC with Differential / Platelet	Result	Flag	Units	Reference Interval
WBC	6.0		x10³/µL	4.0 - 10.5
RBC	5.0		x10⁶/µL	4.1 - 5.6
Hemoglobin	13.0		g/dL	12.5 - 17.0
Hematocrit	45		%	36 - 50
MCV	85		fL	80 - 98
MCH	30		pg	27 - 34
MCHC	34		g/dL	32 - 36
RDW	12.0		%	11.7 - 15
Platelets	200		x10³/µL	140 - 415
Neutrophils	50		%	40 - 74
Lymphocytes	25		%	14 - 46
Monocytes	5		%	4 - 13
Eosinophils	6		%	0 - 7
Basophils	2		%	0 - 3
Neutrophils (absolute)	3.0		x10³/µL	1.8 - 7.8
Lymphocytes (absolute)	1.5		x10³/µL	0.7 - 4.5
Monocytes (absolute)	0.3		x10³/µL	0.1 - 1.0
Eosinophils (absolute)	0.4		x10³/µL	0.0 - 0.4
Basophils (absolute)	0.1		x10³/µL	0.0 - 0.2
Immature Granulocytes	0		%	0 - 1
Immature Granulocytes (absolute)	0.0		x10³/µL	0.0 - 0.1

To schedule time with a Personal Health Coach, please call 1-877-4HDLABS (1-877-443-5227) or visit us online at www.myhdl.com

Lab Notes:

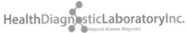
HealthDiagnosticLaboratoryInc.
beyond disease diagnosis

Laboratory Results

NMR LipoProfile® Test

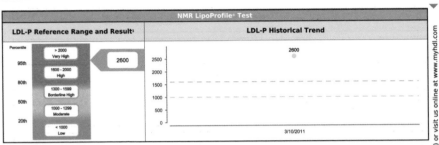

LDL-P Reference Range and Result¹

Percentile	
95th	> 2000 Very High
	1600 - 2000 High
80th	1300 - 1599 Borderline High
50th	1000 - 1299 Moderate
20th	
	< 1000 Low

2600

LDL-P Historical Trend

2600

3/10/2011

Particle Concentration and Size

Laboratory Test	Result	Percentile in Reference Population²				Previous Results
		Higher CVD Risk			Lower CVD Risk	
HDL-P (total) μmol/L	25.0	low	25th (26.7)	50th (30.5)	75th (34.9) high	
			25			

Small LDL-P and LDL Size are associated with CVD risk, but not after LDL-P is taken into account.

Insulin Resistance   Insulin Sensitive

Lipoprotein Markers Associated with Insulin Resistance and Diabetes Risk

To schedule time with a Personal Health Coach, please call 1-877-4HDLABS (1-877-443-5227) or visit us online at www.myhdi.com

HealthDiagnosticLaboratoryInc. Omega 3 and Omega 6 Fatty Acids Profile
beyond disease diagnosis

Patient

Name: Max Test	Phone #:	Patient ID #:
Fasting Status:	Gender:	Birthdate:	Age:
Height:	Weight:	BMI:	Prev. BMI:

Specimen

Collection Time:	Specimen ID:
Collection Date:	Report Type:
Received Date:	Report Date:

Provider

Requesting Provider:
Client ID:

Laboratory Test	Notes	High Risk	Intermediate Risk	Optimal	High Risk Range	Intermediate Risk Range	Optimal Range	Previous Results
Index HS-Omega-3 Index® (RBC EPA+DHA)ᵃ		3.8			< 4.0%	4.0% - 8.0%	> 8.0%	

Comments:

Your HS-Omega-3 Index is well below the target range of 8%.

The HS-Omega-3 Index is the EPA+DHA content of RBC membranes. Increasing the intake of EPA+DHA by 1 to 2 grams (1,000 - 2,000 mg) per day, from either oily fish or fish oil supplements, should significantly improve the index. The exact amount of EPA+DHA needed will vary person to person. A re-check should be done in 3 - 4 months.

Omega-3 Fatty Acids

Fatty Acids	Range	Current	Previous
Omega-3 Total	0.1% - 14.1%	7.9%	
Alpha-Linolenic (ALA)	0.1% - 0.4%	0.3%	
Docosapentaenoic (DPA)	0.6% - 4.1%	7.4%	
Eicosapentaenoic (EPA)	0.1% - 2.5%	1.2%	
Docosahexaenoic (DHA)	0.1% - 8.4%	4.7%	

Omega-6 Fatty Acids

Fatty Acids	Range	Current	Previous
Omega-6 Total	28.6% - 44.5%	36.9%	
Arachidonic (AA)	10.5% - 23.3%	10.3%	
Linoleic (LA)	4.6% - 21.3%	9.7%	

Other Fatty Acids

Fatty Acids	Range	Current	Previous
cis-Monounsaturated Total	11.5% - 20.5%	12.5%	
Saturated Total	36.6% - 42.0%	40.9%	
Trans Total	<0.1% - 1.8%	2.6%	

Content of EPA+DHA (mg/3 oz serving) in Common Seafoods*

Higher Omega-3	EPA+DHA	Intermediate Omega-3	EPA+DHA	Lower Omega-3	EPA+DHA
Salmon Atlantic, farmed	1825	Swordfish	764	Tuna, Light (canned in water)	230
Herring Atlantic	1712	Rainbow Trout, farmed	744	Halibut	200
Salmon Atlantic	1564	Tuna, Albacore or White (canned in water)	733	Northern Lobster (steamed)	165
Tuna Bluefin	1279	Sockeye Salmon	673	Clams (canned)	150
Salmon Chum	1238	Sea Bass	648	Scallops (steamed)	149
Herring Pickled	1181	Salmon Pink	524	Haddock or Cod	135
Salmon Coho, farmed	1087	Crab Dungeness	501	Mahi-Mahi (dolphin fish)	118
Mackerel (canned)	1046	Alaskan Pollock	433	Tilapia	115
Salmon Coho	900	Crab King	351	Shrimp	87
Oysters (steamed)	850	Walleye	338	Catfish, farmed	76
Sardines (canned in oil)	835	Flat fish (Flounder/sole)	255	Orange Roughy	26

*From the USDA Nutrient Database (as of 8/24/11) for fish cooked with dry heat unless otherwise noted, and wild unless indicated as farmed.

ᵃThe HS-Omega-3 Index cutpoints are based on Harris and von Shacky, Preventive Medicine 2004;39:212-220

Dr. Joseph P. McConnell | Laboratory Director | CLIA No. 49D1100708 | CAP No. 7224971 | NPI No. 1629209853
©2010 | 737 N. 5th Street Suite 103 | Richmond, Virginia 23219 | Phone: 804.343.2718 | Fax: 804.343.2704   HDL 20.0

To schedule time with a Personal Health Coach, please call 1-877-4HDLABS (1-877-443-5227) or visit us online at www.myhdi.com

Unfortunately, there are a lot of patients like Max who only get a basic cholesterol panel, are told that their results are "pretty good," and are simply placed on a statin drug and sent on their way with the goal of getting their LDL cholesterol down to less than 100 mg/dl, or less than 70 mg/dl if they are very high risk. By getting Max's expanded metabolic panel, we uncovered "hidden" risk for future heart attack. And by looking at these numbers together with his borderline elevated blood sugar, we also uncovered the likelihood that Max had probably been walking around with insulin resistance for years—and insulin resistance leads to heart attacks. In fact, if he continued his current flawed lifestyle, it was only a matter of time before Max developed type-2 diabetes.

Max was motivated to change; after all, he had two daughters, and he needed to be there for them. Since his numbers were the result of an unhealthy lifestyle, the first order of business was to place him on a diet and exercise program that would optimize his blood chemistry and protect him from future heart attacks.

I discussed with Max and his wife the importance of a Mediterranean-style diet, stressing the regular consumption of fresh fruits and vegetables, whole grains, beans, omega-3-rich fish, and other features of heart-healthy nutrition. I encouraged Max to limit red meat consumption to no more than once or twice a month, and to completely avoid processed meat. I even got him to stop drinking regular (cow's) milk and switch to almond milk. After he passed a screening stress test, I started him on a six-week supervised cardiac rehab program. I encouraged Max to purchase a pedometer and strive for ten thousand steps a day. I taught him some simple stress management techniques, and I had him see his dentist for a routine cleaning—something he had not done in years. In short, I took him through all the steps I've shared in this book for the first four weeks!

When he left the hospital, Max had been given the usual medications following a heart attack, namely a statin, an ACE inhibitor,

GO GREEN

Many labs these days color code your lab results, to tell you in a glance if you are at high risk or low risk for a heart attack. In order to become Heart Attack Proof, it is important to "go green"— that is, move your lab values from yellow (intermediate risk) or red (high risk) to green (optimal). Using lifestyle changes and medical therapy (if necessary) to change these values is your best insurance against a heart attack or stroke.

a beta blocker, and daily aspirin. Due to the extensive nature of his metabolic abnormalities and the fact that he'd already had a heart attack, I switched him to a more potent statin, while continuing his other medications. In view of his low vitamin D level, I started him on a daily vitamin D supplement and I also gave him fish oil supplements to correct his low omega-3 level.

In six months, Max had lost twenty-five pounds and his BMI was normal. Repeat lab work revealed almost a complete resolution of his previously noted metabolic abnormalities:

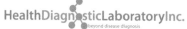

HealthDiagnosticLaboratoryInc.
beyond disease diagnosis

Laboratory Results

Patient

Name: Max Test
Phone #:
Patient ID #:

Fasting Status:
Gender:
Birthdate:
Age:

Height:
Weight:
BMI:
Prev. BMI:

Specimen

Collection Time:
Specimen ID:

Collection Date:
Report Type:

Received Date:
Report Date:

Provider

Requesting Provider:

Client ID:

Laboratory Test	Notes	High Risk	Intermediate Risk	Optimal	High Risk Range	Intermediate Risk Range	Optimal Range	Previous Results 3/10/2011
Lipids								
Total Cholesterol (mg/dL)				128	≥ 240	200 - 239	< 200	156
LDL-C Direct (mg/dL)				48	≥ 130 CHD & CHD risk eq. > 100	100 - 129 CHD & CHD risk eq. 70 - 100	< 100 CHD & CHD risk eq. < 70	73
HDL-C (mg/dL)				45	< 40		≥ 40	35
Triglycerides (mg/dL)				135	≥ 200	150 - 199	< 150	175
Non-HDL-C (mg/dL) (calculated)				83	≥ 160	130 - 159	< 130	121
Lipoprotein Particles and Apolipoproteins								
Apo B (mg/dL)			64		≥ 80	60 - 79	< 60	125
LDL-P (nmol/L)				880	≥ 1300	1000 - 1299	< 1000	2600
sdLDL (mg/dL)*				19	≥ 31	21 - 30	≤ 20	38
Apo A-I (mg/dL)				134	< 114	114 - 131	≥ 132	92
HDL-P (µmol/L)				42.0	< 28.0	28.0 - 34.0	≥ 35.0	25.0
HDL2 (mg/dL)*				14	≤ 8	9 - 11	≥ 12	8
Apo B:Apo A-I Ratio (calculated)				0.48	≥ 0.81	0.61 - 0.81	≤ 0.6	1.36
Lp(a) Mass (mg/dL)				21	≥ 30		< 30	22
Lp(a) Cholesterol (mg/dL)					≥ 6	3 - 5	< 3	
Inflammation/ Oxidation								
Myeloperoxidase (pmol/L)				359	≥ 550	400 - 549	< 400	552
Lp-PLA₂ (ng/mL)				190	> 235	200 - 235	< 200	285
hs-CRP (mg/L)				0.8	≥ 3.0	1.0 - 2.9	< 1.0	2.8
Fibrinogen (mg/dL)					≥ 465	391 - 464	≤ 390	
Myocardial Stress								
NT-proBNP (pg/mL)					≥ 450	125 - 449	< 125	
Platelets								
AspirinWorks® (urine) (pg/mg of creatinine)					> 1500		≤ 1500	

Lab Notes:

Provider Notes:

www.myhdl.com

To schedule time with a Personal Health Coach, please call 1-877-4HDLABS (1-877-443-5227) or visit us online at www.myhdl.com

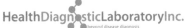

HealthDiagnosticLaboratoryInc.
beyond disease diagnosis

Laboratory Results

To schedule time with a Personal Health Coach, please call 1-877-4HDLABS (1-877-443-5227) or visit us online at www.myhdl.com

Patient
Name: **Max Test**	Phone #:	Patient ID #:
Fasting Status:	Gender:	Birthdate:	Age:
Height:	Weight:	BMI:	Prev. BMI:

Specimen
Collection Time:	Specimen ID:
Collection Date:	Report Type:
Received Date:	Report Date:

Provider
Requesting Provider:
Client ID:

Laboratory Test	Notes	High Risk	Intermediate Risk	Optimal	High Risk Range	Intermediate Risk Range	Optimal Range	Previous Results 3/10/2011
Lipoprotein Genetics								
Apolipoprotein E Genotype*					Estimated Genotype Frequency: 2/2 (~1-2%), 2/3 (~15%), 2/4 (~1-2%), 3/3 (~55%), 3/4 (~25%), 4/4 (~1-2%)			
Platelet Genetics								
CYP2C19*2*3* **POOR** metabolizers with poor antiplatelet effect of Plavix.					*1/*1 = optimal, *1/*2 or *1/*3 = intermediate, *2/*2, *2/*3 or *3/*3 = poor			
CYP2C19*17* **RAPID** metabolizers at increased risk for bleeding on Plavix.					*1/*1 = optimal, *1/*17 = rapid, *17/*17 = ultra rapid			
Coagulation Genetics								
Factor V Leiden					**Optimal**=Non-carrier (Arg/Arg); **At Risk**=(Arg/Gln or Gln/Gln)			
Prothrombin Mutation					**Optimal**=Non-carrier (G/G); **At Risk**=(G/A or A/A)			
Metabolic								
Insulin (µU/mL)					≥ 12	10 - 11	3 - 9	
Free Fatty Acid (mmol/L)					> 0.7	0.6 - 0.7	≤ 0.59	
Glucose (mg/dL)				88	≤ 55 or > 125	56-69 or 100-125	70 - 99	106
HbA1c (%)				5.5	≥ 6.5	5.7 - 6.4	≤ 5.6	6.2
Estimated Average Glucose (mg/dL) (calculated)				111.2	≥ 139.9	116.9 - 139.8	≤ 116.8	131.2
25-hydroxy-Vitamin D (ng/mL)				42	≤ 14	15 - 29	30 - 100	11
TSH (µIU/mL)				2.45	< 0.27 or > 4.20		0.27 - 4.20	2.43
Homocysteine (µmol/L)					> 13	11 - 13	≤ 10	
RBC Folate (ng/mL)				775	≤ 467		≥ 468	
Renal								
Creatinine, serum (mg/dL)				1.1	> 1.2		0.7 - 1.2	1.2

Lab Notes:

Dr. Joseph P. McConnell | Laboratory Director | CLIA No. 49D1100708 | CAP No. 7224971 | NPI No. 1629209853
©2010 | 737 N. 5th Street Suite 103 | Richmond, Virginia 23219 | Phone: 804.343.2718 | Fax: 804.343.2704

HDL 20.0

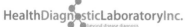

HealthDiagnosticLaboratoryInc.
beyond disease diagnosis

Laboratory Results

Patient

Name: Max Test	Phone #:		Patient ID #:
Fasting Status:	Gender:	Birthdate:	Age:
Height:	Weight:	BMI:	Prev. BMI:

Specimen

Collection Time:	Specimen ID:
Collection Date:	Report Type:
Received Date:	Report Date:

Provider

| Requesting Provider: |
| Client ID: |

Other Biomarkers	Result	Flag	Reference Interval
Albumin (g/dl)	3.7		3.5 - 5.2
ALP (U/L)	110		40 - 129
ALT / GPT (U/L)	38		Up to 41
AST / GOT (U/L)	32		Up to 40
BUN (mg/dl)	14		6 - 20
Calcium (mg/dL)	8.9		8.6 - 10.2
Cl- (mmol/L)	99		96 - 108
CO_2 (mmol/L)	23		22 - 29
K+ (mmol/L)	4.5		3.3 - 5.1
Na+ (mmol/L)	140		133 - 145
Total Bilirubin (mg/dL)	1.1		Up to 1.2
Total Protein (g/dL)	7.2		6.4 - 8.3
T4 (µg/dL)	11.3		4.5 - 11.7
T3 (ng/dL)	154		80 - 200

CBC with Differential / Platelet	Result	Flag	Units	Reference Interval
WBC	9.2		x10³/µL	4.0 - 10.5
RBC	4.3		x10⁶/µL	4.1 - 5.6
Hemoglobin	15.0		g/dL	12.5 - 17.0
Hematocrit	40		%	36 - 50
MCV	85		fL	80 - 98
MCH	28		pg	27 - 34
MCHC	33		g/dL	32 - 36
RDW	11.9		%	11.7 - 15
Platelets	145		x10³/µL	140 - 415
Neutrophils	70		%	40 - 74
Lymphocytes	41		%	14 - 46
Monocytes	5		%	4 - 13
Eosinophils	2		%	0 - 7
Basophils	2		%	0 - 3
Neutrophils (absolute)	6.4		x10³/µL	1.8 - 7.8
Lymphocytes (absolute)	3.8		x10³/µL	0.7 - 4.5
Monocytes (absolute)	0.5		x10³/µL	0.1 - 1.0
Eosinophils (absolute)	0.2		x10³/µL	0.0 - 0.4
Basophils (absolute)	0.2		x10³/µL	0.0 - 0.2
Immature Granulocytes	0		%	0 - 1
Immature Granulocytes (absolute)	0.0	.	x10³/µL	0.0 - 0.1

To schedule time with a Personal Health Coach, please call 1-877-4HDLABS (1-877-443-5227) or visit us online at www.myhdi.com

Lab Notes:

Dr. Joseph P. McConnell | Laboratory Director | CLIA No. 49D1100708 | CAP No. 7224971 | NPI No. 1629209853
©2010 | 737 N. 5th Street Suite 103 | Richmond, Virginia 23219 | Phone: 804.343.2718 | Fax: 804.343.2704

HDL 20.0

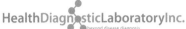
HealthDiagnosticLaboratoryInc.
beyond disease diagnosis

Laboratory Results

Patient	Name: Max Test	Phone #:	Patient ID #:
	Fasting Status:	Gender:	Birthdate:	Age:
	Height:	Weight:	BMI:	Prev. BMI:

Specimen	Collection Time:	Specimen ID:
	Collection Date:	Report Type:
	Received Date:	Report Date:

| Provider | Requesting Provider: |
| | Client ID: |

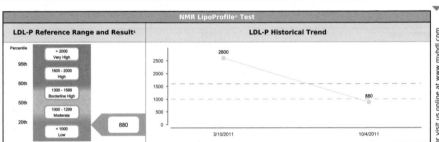

NMR LipoProfile® Test

LDL-P Reference Range and Result[1]

Percentile
95th — > 2000 Very High
80th — 1600 - 2000 High
— 1300 - 1599 Borderline High
50th — 1000 - 1299 Moderate
20th — < 1000 Low

◄ 880

LDL-P Historical Trend

2600 ... 880

3/10/2011   10/4/2011

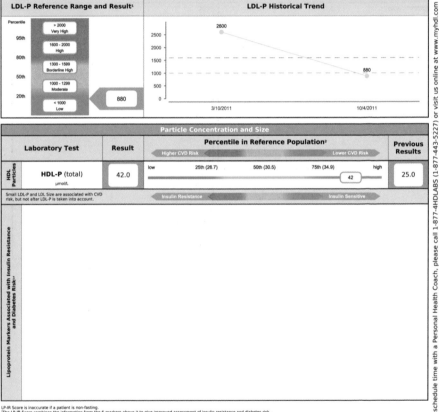

Particle Concentration and Size

Laboratory Test	Result	Percentile in Reference Population[2]				Previous Results
		Higher CVD Risk			Lower CVD Risk	
HDL Particles **HDL-P (total)** µmol/L	42.0	low	25th (26.7)	50th (30.5)	75th (34.9) 42 high	25.0

Small LDL-P and LDL Size are associated with CVD risk, but not after LDL-P is taken into account.

Insulin Resistance ————————————— Insulin Sensitive

Lipoprotein Markers Associated with Insulin Resistance and Diabetes Risk[3]

LP-IR Score is inaccurate if a patient is non-fasting.
'The LP-IR Score combines the information from the 6 markers above it to give improved assessment of insulin resistance and diabetes risk.

These laboratory assays, validated by LipoScience, have not been cleared by the US Food and Drug Administration. The clinical utility of these laboratory values has not been fully established.
1. Reference population comprises '5,362' men and women not on lipid medication enrolled in the Multi-Ethnic Study of Atherosclerosis (MESA). Mora, et al. *Atherosclerosis* 2007.
2. LipoScience reference population comprises 4,588 men and women without known CVD or diabetes and not on lipid medication.
3. Garvey WT, et al. *Diabetes*. 2003; 532:453-462. 4. Goff DC et al. *Metabolism*. 2005; 54:264-270.

Dr. Joseph P. McConnell | Laboratory Director | CLIA No. 49D1100708 | CAP No. 7224971 | NPI No. 1629209853
©2010 | 737 N. 5th Street Suite 103 | Richmond, Virginia 23219 | Phone: 804.343.2718 | Fax: 804.343.2704   HDL 20.0

To schedule time with a Personal Health Coach, please call 1-877-4HDLABS (1-877-443-5227) or visit us online at www.myhdl.com

HealthDiagnosticLaboratoryInc. Omega 3 and Omega 6 Fatty Acids Profile
beyond disease diagnosis

Patient

Name: **Max Test**	Phone #:	Patient ID #:
Fasting Status:	Gender:	Birthdate:	Age:
Height:	Weight:	BMI:	Prev. BMI:

Specimen

Collection Time:	Specimen ID:
Collection Date:	Report Type:
Received Date:	Report Date:

Provider

Requesting Provider:	
Client ID:	

	Laboratory Test	Notes	High Risk	Intermediate Risk	Optimal	High Risk Range	Intermediate Risk Range	Optimal Range	Previous Results 3/10/2011
Index	HS-Omega-3 Index® (RBC EPA+DHA)[a]				8.2	< 4.0%	4.0% - 8.0%	> 8.0%	3.8

Omega-3 Fatty Acids			
Fatty Acids	Range	Current	Previous
Omega-3 Total	0.1% - 14.1%	**7.0%**	7.9%
Alpha-Linolenic (ALA)	0.1% - 0.4%	< 0.1%	0.3%
Docosapentaenoic (DPA)	0.6% - 4.1%	3.2%	7.4%
Eicosapentaenoic (EPA)	0.1% - 2.5%	0.9%	1.2%
Docosahexaenoic (DHA)	0.1% - 8.4%	2.9%	4.7%

Omega-6 Fatty Acids			
Fatty Acids	Range	Current	Previous
Omega-6 Total	28.6% - 44.5%	**33.3%**	36.9%
Arachidonic (AA)	10.5% - 23.3%	11.5%	10.3%
Linoleic (LA)	4.6% - 21.3%	4.9%	9.7%

Other Fatty Acids			
Fatty Acids	Range	Current	Previous
cis-Monounsaturated Total	11.5% - 20.5%	**13.2%**	12.5%
Saturated Total	36.6% - 42.0%	**37.8%**	40.9%
Trans Total	<0.1% - 1.8%	**1.2%**	2.6%

[a]The HS-Omega-3 Index cutpoints are based on Harris and von Shacky, Preventive Medicine 2004;39:212-220

Dr. Joseph P. McConnell | Laboratory Director | CLIA No. 49D1100708 | CAP No. 7224971 | NPI No. 1629209853
©2010 | 737 N. 5th Street Suite 103 | Richmond, Virginia 23219 | Phone: 804.343.2718 | Fax: 804.343.2704   HDL 20.0

When Max looked at his new numbers he had tears in his eyes. He told me that he now felt in control of his life and his destiny. Every day that he looked at his wife and daughters, he realized how lucky he was to be alive and well.

It's been several years since Max had his heart attack. He remains healthy and his blood chemistries have remained normal—including his LDL particle number. Most importantly, Max is happy and confident. He battled the enemy called cardiovascular disease and he slew the monster! He recently walked one of his daughters down the aisle—one of the happiest days of his life.

The Genesis of a Heart Attack

Having these tests done regularly is crucially important. The next step is to understand what all the numbers mean. To do so, we first need to take a step back and look at the development and progression of cardiovascular disease, and how metabolic abnormalities can lead to a heart attack.

A heart attack occurs when the blood supply to the heart is cut off. We used to think that heart attacks were caused by the buildup of cholesterol and fat that ultimately choked off the artery causing a heart attack; we now know that the culprit is not cholesterol itself but the particles that carry it.

There are two types of these particles, characterized by the protein on their surfaces. The first type contains an apoB protein on the surface, which means they have the potential to enter the artery wall and lead to atherosclerotic plaque formation. Ninety percent of particles with apoB proteins are LDL particles. LDL particles are often referred to as "bad" particles, though they are not always bad. They play a beneficial role—they deliver cholesterol throughout the body where it is needed (cholesterol is an essential component of cell membranes, and is also necessary for the body

WHY DO LDL PARTICLES ENTER THE ARTERY WALL?

In nature there is a normal flow from high concentration to low concentration. When the concentration of LDL particles in the bloodstream is high, it is more likely that they will leave the bloodstream and enter the artery wall.

to produce hormones such as cortisol, aldosterone, estrogen, and testosterone, as well as bile acids and vitamin D). But they also have the potential to enter the arterial wall and wreak havoc. The second type is HDL particles. These have a different protein on their surface called apoA1. HDL particles are often referred to as "good" cholesterol particles, because their job is to enter the arterial wall, remove cholesterol, and carry it to the liver for processing.

So, in short, LDL's job is to carry cholesterol to the areas of the body where it's needed, and HDL's job is to pick up excess cholesterol inside the artery wall from the places it isn't needed. All of this is necessary for proper functioning of the body. Problems arise when there is an excess number of LDL particles in the blood and these particles enter the artery wall. Once there, the particles can lead to the formation of atherosclerotic plaques, which are like pimples in the blood vessel wall. And just like pimples, these plaques can become inflamed and rupture.

The Myth of the 90 Percent Blockage

Most plaques that rupture and cause heart attacks are not the large blockages that obstruct the flow of blood in the coronary artery by 80 or 90 percent. The restriction of blood flow in these cases often doesn't lead to a heart attack, as our bodies have methods of rerouting blood flow through collateral channels as these large plaques grow. The real problem is the smaller, highly inflamed plaques that may only narrow the artery by 10 to 50 percent. When these rupture, the artery can become 100 percent blocked in a matter of seconds, which doesn't give the body time to compensate. Blood flow is completely obstructed, and the result is a heart attack. That's why most people who suffer fatal heart attacks, like Tim Russert, have no prior warning. One moment blood is flowing normally; the next, it isn't.

So what causes atherosclerotic plaques to form, and then to rupture? The answer has to do with free radicals and inflammation.

The Formation of Atherosclerotic Plaques

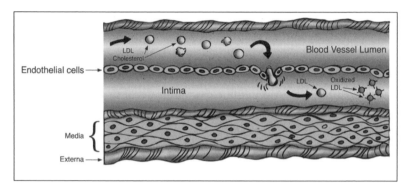

Figure 1. LDL (bad) cholesterol particles squeeze through the lining of the artery wall, where the cholesterol is retained and becomes oxidized.

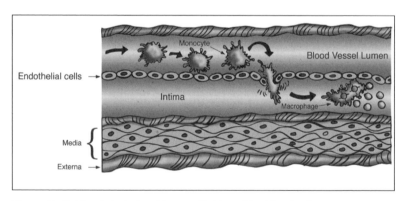

Figure 2. Oxidized cholesterol is engulfed by white blood cells.

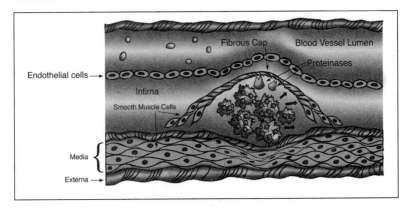

Figure 3. The plaque develops a thick fibrous cap, which is attacked by proteinases.

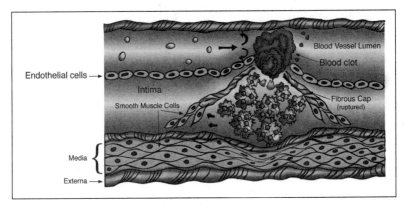

Figure 4. The fibrous cap breaks down. When blood enters the plaque, it comes into contact with tissue factor and activates platelets, which cause the blood to clot and block flow in the artery.

Once inside the artery wall, cholesterol particles come into contact with something called *free radicals*. *Free radical* is the term used for any molecule with an uneven number of electrons. You may remember from chemistry class that molecules with uneven numbers of electrons don't like to stay that way. They'll do whatever they can to beg, borrow, or steal another electron so they can have an even number. This theft by free radicals is referred to as *oxidation*.

When a free radical steals an electron from a cholesterol-carrying particle, the particle then becomes oxidized, and the body views it as a foreign invader. As a result, our natural defense system—inflammation—kicks in. Our immune system goes on the attack and sends white blood cells to the scene to engulf the oxidized cholesterol particles, and this leads to the formation of an atherosclerotic plaque.

After engulfing the cholesterol particles, the white blood cells, called *macrophages*, begin to release proteinases, which are designed to break down the plaque's fibrous cap, ultimately causing the plaque to rupture. When blood comes into contact with tissue factor (a clot-promoting molecule) inside the plaque, it forms a clot at the rupture site. If that clot is large enough, it can completely block the artery, leading to a heart attack.

Reversing Heart Disease

As you can see, there are a number of complex factors at work in causing a heart attack. The good news is, it's possible to not only halt the progression of atherosclerosis, but to *actually reverse it*.

With the proper lifestyle and optimal medical therapy, it is possible to stabilize and even get rid of the atherosclerotic plaques that lead to heart attacks. As we've learned more about how plaque formation and rupture works, we've realized that regression of atherosclerosis is an achievable goal.

A recent study of the statin medication Crestor (rosuvastatin) showed this in action. In 507 patients with measurable coronary artery disease, Crestor, which significantly lowered LDL (bad) cholesterol and raised HDL (good) cholesterol, also resulted in a decrease in the size of the patients' atherosclerotic plaque.

So let's get started! We'll take the results of your blood tests category by category, discuss what they measure and why that's important, and then go over what you can do to bring your results into the optimal range. It may just save your life!

Cholesterol

When I started my cardiology practice in 1979, a normal cholesterol level was up to 300 mg/dl! Today we know better. It is now recommended that your cholesterol level should remain under 200 mg/dl (see the National Cholesterol Education Panel's official cholesterol guidelines in Appendix E). And thanks to research like the Framingham Study, we know the optimal total cholesterol is actually less than 150 mg/dl. Yet the average total cholesterol for Americans is still greater than 200 mg/dl (208 mg/dl).

As we saw with Max, knowing your total cholesterol is an important part of understanding your risk for a heart attack. But it doesn't always tell the whole story of what's happening inside your body. To get the rest, you need to look at several other factors—in particular, non-HDL cholesterol, LDL and HDL particle numbers, and triglycerides.

THE 150 CLUB

Dr. William Castelli, a noted preventive cardiologist and former director of the Framingham Study, frequently mentioned the "150 club" when talking about the study's results. He noted that none of the study subjects with a total cholesterol less than 150 mg/dl had suffered a heart attack. Other studies supported what the Framingham Study had found—populations around the world with practically nonexistent coronary heart disease and heart attack had average total cholesterol between 120 and 150.

Non-HDL Cholesterol

Non-HDL cholesterol is just what it sounds like: the amount of cholesterol in your blood not contained in HDL particles. It's calculated by taking your total cholesterol and subtracting your HDL cholesterol from it—in essence, subtracting the good cholesterol from total cholesterol to give you a number that reflects the total amount of bad cholesterol contained in particles that can potentially enter the arterial wall and lead to atherosclerosis.

This measurement is not the same as LDL cholesterol. Ninety percent of bad-cholesterol-carrying particles are LDL particles, but there are other particles that can potentially carry bad cholesterol, including VLDL, IDL, LPa, and chylomicrons. So a measurement of non-HDL cholesterol turns out to be a better reflection of cardiovascular risk than measuring LDL cholesterol alone, since it checks the amount of cholesterol in *all* of the potentially bad particles. Non-HDL cholesterol is especially useful when triglyceride levels are elevated.

The following example shows how easily non-HDL can be calculated. Let's say we're looking at the following routine cholesterol panel:

Total cholesterol: 156 mg/dl
LDL cholesterol: 80 mg/dl
HDL cholesterol: 40 mg/dl
Triglycerides: 180 mg/dl

This person's non-HDL cholesterol is his or her total cholesterol (156 mg/dl) minus HDL cholesterol (40 mg/dl)—or 116 mg/dl.

A normal non-HDL cholesterol is less than 130 mg/dl. However, a value of less than 100 mg/dl is advised for those men and women who are at high risk for cardiovascular disease.

Particle Number

The next important factor in heart attack prevention—possibly the most important factor—is your particle number. Decreasing the number of (bad) LDL particles in your blood and increasing the number of (good) HDL particles is key.

Remember, cholesterol is transported through the bloodstream by particles, and atherosclerotic plaques occur when LDL particles enter the artery wall, get retained, and become oxidized. You can think of the particles as cars and cholesterol molecules as passengers in the cars. Just as too many cars can cause a traffic jam, too many LDL particles can lead to a heart attack. It is the number of particles, not the amount of cholesterol in the particles, that is the problem.

Since the cholesterol content of LDL particles is variable, LDL particle number (LDL-P) is a better measure of future heart attack risk than LDL cholesterol (LDL-C). This explains how someone could have a heart attack despite having a "normal" cholesterol level; measuring cholesterol tells us the amount of cholesterol being carried but not the number of particles doing the carrying.

An increased number of LDL particles, whether those particles are large or small, will increase the risk of a heart attack (studies have shown that an increased number of small particles raises heart attack risk sixfold, whereas an increased number of large particles raises risk twofold). The likelihood of LDL particles entering the arterial wall is largely a function of LDL particles' concentration in the bloodstream; fewer LDL particles means fewer LDL particles entering the artery wall. Men and women who are overweight or

PARTICLES PREDICT DISEASE

Recent scientific studies have shown that it is the number of LDL particles, not the amount of cholesterol carried in those particles, that is the best predictor of future heart attack risk.

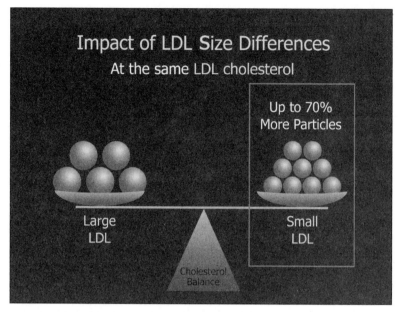

Figure 5. Two people with the same level of cholesterol may have different levels of risk due to the number of particles carrying that cholesterol through their bloodstream.

obese and who have insulin resistance, metabolic syndrome, or diabetes are more likely to have an increased number of small LDL particles, while individuals with familial hyperlipidemia, a genetic disorder, have an excess number of large LDL particles. The key for both groups is to lower the number of excess LDL particles through lifestyle intervention and medication.

Unfortunately, many healthcare providers do not normally measure particle number in addition to cholesterol—even though clinical studies, such as the Framingham Offspring Study, have demonstrated that LDL particle number is a superior predictor of heart attack risk than the measurement of total cholesterol or LDL cholesterol. So be informed, and discuss particle number measurement with your physician.

Triglycerides

The final factor to consider is triglycerides. Triglycerides are a type of fat that, if elevated, can increase cardiovascular risk by increasing the number of small dense LDL particles and decreasing the number of HDL particles. Elevated triglycerides can also lead to pancreatitis (inflammation of the pancreas).

The Optimal Lipid Profile

The chart below lists the recommended and optimal values for a standard lipid profile, including particle number (for both apoB and LDL-P). To become Heart Attack Proof, you want your numbers to be as close to optimal as possible.

	Recommended	Optimal
Total Cholesterol	< 200 mg/dl	< 150 mg/dl
LDL cholesterol	< 100 mg/dl	< 70 mg/dl
HDL cholesterol	> 40 mg/dl (for men) > 50 mg/dl (for women)	> 40 mg/dl (for men) > 50 mg/dl (for women)
Non-HDL Cholesterol	< 130 mg/dl	< 100 mg/dl
Triglycerides	< 150 mg/dl	< 100 mg/dl
LDL-P	< 1000 nmol/L	< 700 nmol/L
apoB	< 90 mg/dl	< 60 mg/dl

Many physicians believe that LDL cholesterol needs to be lowered to optimal levels (less than 70 mg/dl) only if you are at very high risk for coronary heart disease, or you actually have coronary heart disease or have suffered a heart attack. That line of reasoning has never made sense to me. Why wait until you've had a heart attack to lower your LDL cholesterol to optimal levels? Remember, half the men and women who suffer a heart attack have no prior warning, and many don't survive their first event. Why not be

BUILDING A BRICK HOUSE

In order to build a brick house, you must have bricks. Hammers, nails, lumber, and insulation all contribute to the construction of the house, but without bricks—you don't have a brick house! Likewise, in order to have an atherosclerotic plaque, you must have atherogenic (mainly LDL) particles. Inflammation, oxidative stress, high blood pressure, diabetes, and other factors may all contribute to plaque development—but without sufficient LDL particles, you don't develop an atherosclerotic plaque. Not enough bricks—no brick house. Not enough LDL particles—no atherosclerotic plaque.

proactive and lower your total cholesterol, LDL cholesterol, non-HDL cholesterol, and LDL particle number to levels that virtually prevents a heart attack in the first place?

Lowering Your Cholesterol Levels

Since the root cause of atherosclerotic plaque formation is the entry and retention in the artery wall of increased numbers of cholesterol-carrying particles, it stands to reason that the most effective therapy is to lower your total cholesterol and the number of (bad) LDL particles while increasing the number of (good) HDL particles through lifestyle modification and, if necessary, medication.

Our cholesterol comes from two sources: what we eat, and what our body produces on its own. The body needs cholesterol to function normally, so it manufactures cholesterol as needed. However, when we take in excess amounts of cholesterol through our diet, it can cause real problems.

Some individuals have a genetic basis for elevated cholesterol and require aggressive medical therapy to control cholesterol levels

WHEN TO GET YOUR CHOLESTEROL TESTED

The National Cholesterol Education Program recommends that people begin regular cholesterol testing at age twenty (earlier if you have risk factors for heart disease). There is no risk in being tested, so you should consider regular testing even if you are healthy. Learning about your cardiovascular disease risk early in life will allow you to take necessary steps, including dietary and exercise modification, to maintain a healthy heart for a lifetime.

and lower their risk of heart attack. Fortunately, genetic causes of high cholesterol are rare: the odds of having familial heterozygous hyperlipidemia (a genetic disorder associated with a decreased ability to remove LDL cholesterol from the bloodstream) is 1 in 500, and the odds of you having familial homozygous hyperlipidemia (an even more severe type) is 1 in a million. This means that the overwhelming majority of men and women with elevated cholesterol levels have a flawed lifestyle—primarily poor dietary choices and sedentary habits—and therefore have it within their power to achieve optimal cholesterol levels.

The first step to doing so is adopting a diet of nutritious, non-processed foods from the earth and sea—in other words, the Mediterranean diet, which has been proven to lower LDL cholesterol, lower LDL particle number, raise HDL cholesterol, and lower triglyceride levels. You can lower your cholesterol levels by 25 percent or more simply by following a Mediterranean diet.

The top foods that have been shown to have a favorable impact on cholesterol, by lowering LDL (bad) cholesterol or by raising HDL (good) cholesterol, include many discussed in the previous chapter. The fiber in fruits and vegetables lowers cholesterol; in addition, plant sterols in fruits and vegetables interfere with the intestinal absorption of cholesterol. The omega-3s in fish lower triglycerides, and red wine raises HDL cholesterol.

LDL CHOLESTEROL LEVELS—HOW LOW TO GO?

Recent research has shown that, even in the presence of other major risk factors for cardiovascular disease, atherosclerosis does not seem to develop when LDL-cholesterol levels are less than 70 mg/dl, if that number is maintained throughout your lifetime.

A recent study demonstrated the importance of cholesterol-lowering food in our diet. Women who ate one apple a day for a year lowered their LDL cholesterol by 23 percent and raised their HDL cholesterol by 4 percent. In addition, daily apple consumption lowered inflammation and free radicals, thereby lowering heart attack risk.

The second step is to exercise! Exercise has been shown to lower total cholesterol, lower LDL particle number, raise HDL cholesterol, and lower triglycerides, as well as make LDL cholesterol particles larger and potentially less dangerous.

Top cholesterol-lowering foods include:

- Almonds
- Beans
- Cold-water fish (salmon, tuna, sardines)
- Cinnamon
- Flaxseed
- High-fiber fruits and vegetables
- Oatmeal
- Plant stanol or sterol spreads
- Soy protein
- Whole grains

If Your Numbers Are Still Too High

For those whose elevated cholesterol levels persist despite lifestyle intervention, another option is cholesterol-lowering medication. Please note, however, that the decision to begin medication should be discussed with your personal physician, based on your overall risk for developing cardiovascular disease. And medication should only be used in addition to, not as a substitute for, a healthy lifestyle.

If your doctor does decide to put you on cholesterol-lowering medication, there are a couple of popular options. The most effective medications available today are HMG-CoA reductase inhibitors, commonly known as statins. Examples of the more popular statins include simvastatin (Zocor), atorvastatin (Lipitor), and rosuvastatin (Crestor). Statins reduce

Ways to lower your cholesterol:

- Decreasing the consumption of food that contains cholesterol, saturated fat, and trans fat
- Increasing the consumption of food that has been shown to reduce LDL cholesterol, such as oatmeal, high-fiber fruits, and vegetables
- Exercising
- Using cholesterol-lowering medications (when diet and exercise do not get you to your goal)

cholesterol levels by decreasing the production of cholesterol in the body. Clinical trials evaluating the impact of statins on heart disease prevention have demonstrated a significant lowering of heart attack risk and death from coronary heart disease. Niacin, resins, and cholesterol-absorption inhibitors are other choices to help lower cholesterol levels. You can see a list of cholesterol-lowering medications, along with their generic and brand names and details about how they work, in Appendix G. And new medications are currently being developed that enhance the lowering of LDL (bad) cholesterol, raising of HDL (good) cholesterol, lowering of triglycerides, and reduction of inflammation within the artery wall.

Again, let me stress: we must not think of these pharmaceutical agents as replacements for the healthy food and physical activity our bodies need. Medications should be used, if needed, in addition to a healthy lifestyle, not in place of one.

Inflammation

As you now know, inflammation is involved in all stages of coronary artery disease, from the formation of plaque in the artery wall, to the plaque's progression and rupture, to the clot that blocks blood flow to the heart muscle. The more pronounced your body's inflammatory response, the more likely your plaques will form, rupture, and lead to heart attacks or strokes.

CAUTION

Your heart and cardiovascular system are not the only parts of you that are negatively affected by chronic inflammation. Researchers at the Karolinska Institute in Stockholm reported in *Brain, Behavior and Immunity* that, in a study of more than fifty thousand young men, those with low-grade inflammation performed worse on standardized intelligence tests and were more likely to die from a premature death.

Chronic inflammation may also inhibit the release of nitric oxide, the chemical responsible for the dilation of blood vessels, which leads to narrowed arteries, decreased blood flow, and increased blood pressure—all of which make it easier for clots to block the flow of blood.

What is clear is that any inflammatory state that becomes chronic, even on a low-grade level, is hazardous to your health, and doing your best to reduce the cause of the inflammation is important to protecting your heart—and your life.

Testing for Inflammation

The two most commonly used biomarkers of vascular inflammation are hs-CRP and Lp-PLA2. There are many clinical trials around the world showing that both hs-CRP and LpPLA2 predict an increased risk of heart attack and stroke when their levels are elevated. Nevertheless, the two blood tests are complementary, since both together are more predictive of a potential cardiovascular event than either test alone. In fact, elevated LpPLA2 tells us that the risk of stroke is increased fivefold, whereas elevated LpPLA2 and hs-CRP tells us that the risk is increased elevenfold!

The chart below lists the recommended and optimal values for both hs-CRP and Lp-PLA2.

	Recommended	Optimal
hs-CRP	< 2.0 mg/L	< 1.0 mg/L
Lp-PLA2	< 200 ng/ml	< 200 ng/ml

Lowering Elevated hs-CRP and/or Lp-PLA2

Therapeutic options for elevated hs-CRP and/or Lp-PLA2 include lifestyle intervention and medications.

Key lifestyle changes:

- Heart-healthy diet, such as a Mediterranean diet
- Regular exercise
- Smoking cessation
- Weight control

Helpful medications and supplements:

- Statins
- Fish oil
- Niacin
- Fenofibrate
- Ezetimibe
- Aspirin

HOW TO PREVENT AND REVERSE ATHEROSCLEROSIS

- Decrease the number of bad particles that initiate atherosclerosis by achieving optimal levels of apoB and LDL-P.
- Increase the removal of cholesterol from atherosclerotic plaque by achieving optimal levels of HDL.
- Reduce vascular inflammation by achieving optimal levels of hs-CRP and Lp-PLA2.

In addition, research is currently under way evaluating novel inhibitors of CRP and LpPLA2 to determine whether these inhibitors are safe and have clinical outcome benefit—namely, prevention of heart attack and stroke.

The Causes of Chronic Inflammation

Chronic inflammation can be caused by a number of factors. The good news is that a state of chronic inflammation can be lowered or eliminated through a heart-healthy diet and lifestyle changes—the exact ones we have outlined in this six-week plan. If you follow the recommendations outlined in this book, you will significantly reduce chronic inflammation in your body.

Inflammatory Culprit #1: The Typical American Diet

The typical American diet we discussed in Week 1 and Week 4—one that is high in red meat, omega-6 fat, trans fat, and refined sugar, and low in omega-3 fat—promotes inflammation. It does so not only by increasing the consumption of unhealthy, highly processed food, but also by contributing to a state of being overweight or obese and increasing abdominal fat. Fat cells, also called adipose cells, release inflammatory proteins into the bloodstream, putting the body into a chronic state of low-grade inflammation. Don't despair, however. Although the American diet increases inflammation, the Mediterranean diet reduces it—yet another reason to begin a Mediterranean style of eating.

Inflammatory Culprit #2: Chronic Inflammatory Conditions

Chronic inflammatory conditions include:

- Arthritis
- Autoimmune disease
- Bronchitis
- Inflammatory bowel disease
- Obesity
- Periodontal disease
- Prostatitis

Make sure that if you have a chronic inflammatory disease, you are seeing a healthcare professional on a regular basis as well as managing it through a healthy diet, regular exercise, and medications when necessary.

Inflammatory Culprit #3: Environmental Toxins

Our bodies are exposed to numerous microscopic toxins every day, and over time, pesticides, chemicals, food additives, and pollution cause our bodies to react in a defensive way, by mounting an inflammatory response.

Countless epidemiologic studies have found that farmers, migrant workers, and pesticide handlers show increased inflammation. Researchers are also linking environmental pollution to adverse cardiac outcomes like heart attacks. Though these studies have been conducted all over the world, they have all had similar results.

A study published in the *New England Journal of Medicine* looked at cardiovascular events based on exposure to air pollutants in more than 65,000 postmenopausal women who lived in thirty-six metropolitan areas in the United States. The results were conclusive: every

WHAT ABOUT ANTI-INFLAMMATORY MEDICATIONS?

Certain medications that reduce chronic inflammation have been shown to lower the risk of heart attack. Aspirin is an excellent example: besides blocking platelets and lowering the risk of blood clots, it also reduces inflammation by targeting and deactivating specific pro-inflammatory enzymes.

A word of caution, however: most anti-inflammatory medications have adverse cardiovascular side effects, such as raising blood pressure and increasing the risk of heart attack. This includes many over-the-counter anti-inflammatory medications known as NSAIDs (non-steroidal anti-inflammatory drugs), such as ibuprofen. Always discuss the potential risks of these medications with your physician, and try to avoid their chronic use.

---

incremental rise (10 micrograms per cubic meter) in particulate matter—the pollution found in smoke and haze—correlated to a 24 percent increase in the risk of death from cardiovascular disease.

In Mexico City, one of the worst cities in North America in terms of air quality, researchers conducted a post-mortem study of the hearts of twenty-one adolescents and young adults from two different areas of the city. What they found was alarming: the young hearts showed signs of chronic inflammation from exposure to particulate matter as well as endotoxins, microscopic particles of dead bacteria that gain entry to the body by attaching to particulate matter.

A study from Long Island Jewish Medical Center compared twenty-four-hour particulate matter counts in New York City to the number of out-of-hospital cardiac arrests. The researchers reported in the *American Journal of Epidemiology* that on the days when there were rises in small-particle air pollution (despite still falling within "safe" levels as determined by the EPA), there was a 4 to 10 percent increase in the number of heart attacks.

There's even more evidence. Scientists in Germany found that people who live in urban areas where particulate air pollution is high have higher blood pressure than those who live in less polluted areas. And researchers in Boston conducted a study to assess whether particulates in haze, smog, and smoke affected diabetes—a risk factor for cardiovascular disease. The result, published in *Diabetes Care*, was the first ever to show a correlation between type-2 diabetes and air pollution, even after accounting for risk factors such as obesity, exercise, and ethnicity. For every incremental rise in pollution, there was a consistent rise in the prevalence of diabetes.

While it isn't reasonable to expect you to pack up and move away from your urban condo or your house near the highway, it is useful to realize that these environmental pollutants are affecting your health. Doing so means you'll be in a better position to take what steps you can to limit these toxins' effects. Monitor the air quality in your area and avoid exercising outdoors when there is an air quality warning. Avoid contact with pesticides and pollutants. You can even become active in your community to help insure optimal air quality.

Free Radicals

Cholesterol and inflammation are especially key to the progression of heart disease, which is why most of the blood tests we're interested in focus on these. But before we get to the remaining tests, I want to say a few words about another important factor in the development of atherosclerotic plaques: free radicals.

Both the typical American diet and environmental toxins carry another important danger related to cardiovascular health: they cause increased free radical production. When toxins enter your body, whether through your diet or through the air you breathe, they cause free radical production to go into overdrive. Scientists do not know exactly why this happens; we just know that adding unhealthy items to your body is like adding lighter fluid to a fire—the result is a free radical explosion.

Free radicals, you'll recall, are responsible for the oxidation of cholesterol in artery walls, which leads to plaque formation. So the fewer free radicals you have in your body, the lower your risk of developing heart disease.

There is a way to test for free radical and oxidative stress activity in your body, and that's by testing myeloperoxidase. Myeloperoxidase is an enzyme in white blood cells that is elevated in unstable atherosclerotic plaques. This elevated level is associated with a twofold increased risk of heart attack, stroke, or cardiovascular death.

	Recommended	Optimal
Myeloperoxidase (MPO)	< 400 pmol/L	< 400 pmol/L

In our modern, industrial world, it is impossible to get away from toxins altogether, but certain offenders are particularly important to be aware of, as they result in extreme free radical production.

Here's excellent news, however: we know how to fight free radicals. As with many of the risk factors related to heart disease, the damage done by free radicals can be reduced through smart and healthy lifestyle choices. We can abstain from smoking (and choose not to sit close to others who smoke), minimize our exposure to air pollution, and, of course, avoid the highly processed, calorie-dense, and nutrient-depleted American diet that leads to free radical production.

Do you want to create an army of damaging molecules inside your body just because you are craving a hamburger and French fries? I wouldn't! And would you still want the burger and fries if you knew that simply changing your food choices to a healthy fare could create an army of helpful, beneficial molecules inside your body instead?

Your diet is also the key to making free radicals stable and stopping the chain reaction of free radical production—through antioxidants.

Antioxidants: The Antidote to Free Radicals

We've heard a lot in the last few years about antioxidants and their abilities to transform our health for the better. What do they do and what's their benefit?

Toxins to avoid:

- Air pollutants
- Cigarette smoke
- Excess ultraviolet rays from the sun
- Pesticides
- Radiation (especially CAT scans, unless absolutely needed)
- Excessive alcohol
- Preservatives in foods and food packaging
- Industrial chemicals
- Household cleaners

Antioxidants are the body's defense system—they combat and quench the biochemical fires that result from free radical formation. These vitamins and nutrients work by supplying free radicals with the extra electron they would otherwise steal from cholesterol or DNA or other cells. Unlike other molecules, like cholesterol, antioxidants can lose an electron to a free radical without becoming free radicals themselves.

Our bodies create some antioxidant nutrients to help manage the chaos of free radicals. But we need thousands of different antioxidants to remain healthy. The best way to get them is to eat a wide range of fruits and vegetables, in a variety of colors. Why? Because fruits and vegetables are literally color-coded—you can tell what kind of antioxidants they contain by the color of their skin and fruit! So the wider the range of different-colored food you eat, the wider the variety of free radical-fighting antioxidants you'll get.

COLOR YOUR PLATE!

Filling your plate with a rainbow of colors will mean that you are getting a good selection of different antioxidants. Here's a list of great fruits and vegetables and their protective antioxidants, by color:

Orange	Oranges (vitamin C)
	Carrots (beta-carotene, pectin)
	Sweet potatoes/yams (beta-carotene, dioscorin)
Red	Tomatoes (vitamin C, lycopene)
	Apples (quercetin)
	Beets (pectin)
Blue	Blueberries (flavonoids, ellagic acid anthocyanin, vitamin E)
Green	Broccoli (indole-3-carbinol, sulforaphane)
	Asparagus (folate, b vitamins, glutathione)
	Spinach (beta-carotene, lutein, zeaxanthin, flavonoids)
White	Garlic (allicin, diallyl disulphide)
	Cauliflower (glucosinolates, quercetin, vitamin K, sulforaphane)

Recently, research has exploded with study after study looking at specific nutrients in foods with antioxidant properties.

Resveratrol, the potent plant-based antioxidant found in grapes and wine, continues to show promise. Endocrinologists at the University of Buffalo conducted a prospective human trial of resveratrol's ability to control oxidative stress and inflammation in the body. The results, which were published in the *Journal of Clinical Endocrinology & Metabolism*, showed that 40 mg of resveratrol daily suppressed the generation of free radicals when compared to

TAP INTO THE POWER OF ANTIOXIDANTS WITH A MEDITERRANEAN DIET

One of the reasons the Mediterranean diet is so powerful is that it includes so many foods that are antioxidant-rich. Below are just a few examples!

---

a placebo pill. Blood samples from those receiving the antioxidant also showed reduced levels of inflammatory markers, such as inflammatory tumor necrosis factor (TNF) and other inflammatory proteins.

The benefits of resveratrol were demonstrated in another intriguing experiment reported in the *Journal of the Federation of American Societies for Experimental Biology*. One group of subjects was given a simple meal of turkey cutlets, while a second group received the turkey cutlets plus 200 mL (about 6.8 fluid ounces) of resveratrol-rich red wine. A third group was given turkey cutlets that had been soaked in red wine before cooking plus the glass of red wine.

When the researchers measured the participants' blood for markers of oxidative stress after the meal, both the first and second groups had produced free radicals. But the third group had reduced their marker levels to *zero*! This experiment also highlighted a simple concept: by consuming even ordinary foods, such as turkey, our bodies inevitably produce free radicals...unless there are plenty of antioxidants ingested during the same meal.

Food	Antioxidant
Red wine	Resveratrol
Green tea	Catechins
Pomegranate	Ellagitannins
Muscadine grape	Resveratrol
Turmeric	Curcuminoids

Other Important Numbers

In addition to cholesterol and inflammation biomarkers, there are four other key numbers to look at: your blood pressure, your fasting blood sugar, and your omega-3 and vitamin D levels.

Blood Pressure

Your blood pressure is the measure of the force of your blood against the artery wall. The first number in your blood pressure reading, the *systolic pressure*, is the pressure exerted on the artery wall as your heart beats; the second number, the *diastolic pressure*, is the pressure exerted as your heart relaxes between beats. Less than 140/90 mmHg used to be considered a normal blood pressure reading, with 120/80 mmHg as ideal. But after some recent changes, the guidelines now list normal as less than 120/80 mmHg. Blood pressure between 120/80 and 140/90 is now considered pre-hypertension, and anything above 140/90 is considered hypertension (or high blood pressure).

	Optimal	Pre-hypertension	Hypertension
Blood pressure	< 120/80 mm/hg	120/80–140/90 mm/hg	> 140/90 mm/hg

It is normal for your blood pressure to fluctuate during the day due to physical activity or stressful stimuli. However, it should return to normal as your body adjusts to whatever situation you're in. If it doesn't adjust—if, instead, it remains chronically elevated above 140/90 mmHg—you will likely be diagnosed with hypertension.

Hypertension is quite common; it affects more than 50 million Americans. And it can have many causes, the primary one being aging. As we age, blood vessels lose their elasticity, causing a

HOLD THE SODIUM!

Sodium is an essential electrolyte, but it is necessary only in moderate amounts. Hunter-gatherer populations, who had exceptional cardiovascular profiles, consumed a fraction of the sodium modern humans do today. Excessive sodium intake directly affects blood pressure, leading to hypertension. Consuming too much sodium causes the kidneys to retain water, also pushing blood pressure up. Because of this, the American Heart Association recommends that the average person limit their sodium intake to less than 2,300 mg per day, and less than 1500 mg per day for those at increased risk of cardiovascular disease. I recommend that most men and women should limit sodium consumption; remember, one teaspoon of table salt has 2,000 mg of sodium. As always, check with your healthcare provider before making any changes.

decrease in their ability to expand and contract. A young, healthy artery reacts like a balloon when under pressure—it expands. But older arteries aren't flexible enough to expand, so the blood creates greater force against the artery wall as it moves through, leading to a rise in systolic blood pressure. Increased systolic blood pressure is a key indicator of stroke, especially in the elderly.

Another common cause of hypertension is genetics: some people are more predisposed to having high blood pressure than others. But if that's you, it just means that making lifestyle choices that lower your blood pressure—like proper diet, exercise, and not smoking—is even more important.

Hypertension that is largely preventable, or caused by treatable conditions, is called secondary hypertension, meaning it is the result of something else. At this point, you may not be surprised to learn that one of the most common treatable conditions responsible

Control blood pressure the natural way:

- Limit sodium (< 1500 mg/day)
- Consume a wide variety of fruits and vegetables
- Drink grape and pomegranate juice
- Exercise daily
- Stop smoking
- Avoid trans fat
- Avoid excess alcohol
- Avoid excess caffeine
- Manage stress
- Achieve an ideal body weight
- Treat sleep apnea (if present)

for hypertension is poor nutrition. For example, excessive salt intake or too much alcohol or caffeine can cause elevated blood pressure. One question I always ask my patients with hypertension is whether they eat licorice. Licorice contains glycyrrhizin, a substance that can cause sodium retention and drive up blood pressure.

Men and women who have a chronically elevated blood pressure have an increased risk of heart attack, stroke, peripheral vascular disease, and kidney disease. Treatment of high blood pressure can lower cardiovascular risk and should always start with lifestyle intervention; if that doesn't control blood pressure, anti-hypertension medications can be added.

There are a variety of medications that are used to lower blood pressure. Examples of the more common include:

- Angiotension converting enzyme (ACE) inhibitors
- Angiotension receptor blockers (ARBs)
- Thiazide diuretics
- Calcium channel blockers
- Beta blockers

Blood Sugar

When we eat, carbohydrates in our food are broken down and enter the bloodstream as glucose (sugar) to supply the body with energy. The body regulates the glucose levels in the blood by releasing insulin from the pancreas. Normal fasting glucose is less than 100 mg/dl, 100 to 125 mg/dl is considered impaired fasting glucose (pre-diabetes), and a fasting glucose greater than 125 mg/dl indicates diabetes.

Symptoms of diabetes may include:

- Increased thirst
- Increased hunger
- Weight loss or gain
- Frequent urination
- Fatigue or exhaustion
- Delayed healing of cuts or sores
- Blurred vision

When you went to the doctor in Week 1, you had your blood sugar tested to check for diabetes. In addition to measuring your fasting blood sugar, your doctor should have measured your hemoglobin A1c (HbA1c) as a way of checking your average blood sugar level. Normal levels of glucose produce a normal amount of glycated hemoglobin. As the average blood sugar increases, HbA1c increases as well. Therefore HbA1c can indicate your average blood glucose levels over the previous month. High levels of HgA1c reflect poor blood sugar (glucose) control and are associated with an increased risk of cardiovascular disease, nephropathy, and retinopathy. In 2010, the American Diabetes Association added an HgA1c greater than or equal to 6.5 percent as another criteria for the diagnosis of diabetes. Optimal HbA1c is less than 5.7 percent.

	Normal	Impaired fasting glucose	Diabetes
Fasting blood sugar (FBS)	< 100 mg/dl	100–125 mg/dl	> 125 mg/dl

	Optimal	Intermediate risk	Diabetes
Hemoglobin A1c (HbA1c)	< 5.7%	5.7–6.4%	> 6.4%

There are three main types of diabetes:

- *Type-1 diabetes.* Type-1 diabetes usually appears in childhood or adolescence and is characterized by a defect in the cells of the pancreas that manufacture insulin. This type of diabetes is generally believed to be related to autoimmune factors or possibly a virus.
- *Type-2 diabetes.* Type-2 diabetes usually appears in adults and is caused by insulin resistance (in which cells become resistant or less responsive to insulin). This type of diabetes has been increasing worldwide and is believed to be caused by poor diet, lack of exercise, and weight gain. Regrettably, we are now seeing overweight children and adolescents with type-2 diabetes as a result of the toxic American diet and lack of exercise.
- *Gestational diabetes.* Gestational diabetes usually appears in the mother during pregnancy and goes away on its own after the child's birth. It does require active monitoring, however, for the safety of both mother and baby.

All types of diabetes, regardless of cause, have been shown to increase the risk of cardiovascular disease.

Why Insulin Is So Important

Insulin is a hormone produced by specialized cells in the pancreas, and it plays a crucial role in allowing our cells to process sugar. In essence, insulin works like a key, "unlocking" cells and allowing glucose inside, where it can be used as an energy source or stored as glycogen. Without insulin, glucose remains in the bloodstream, and cells aren't able to receive the energy they need to survive and perform necessary functions in our body.

In the case of type-2 diabetes, it's as if someone gummed up the locks so the key no longer fits; insulin no longer opens up cells to receive glucose as efficiently. As a result, the body increases its insulin production to get the cells the glucose they need, and over time, the cells in the pancreas that produce the insulin just burn out. The result is higher levels of blood glucose.

Elevated blood glucose levels can lead to advanced glycation end products (AGEs) in the blood vessel wall. These AGEs stimulate inflammatory cells to release proteinases, which can further weaken the fibrous cap of atherosclerotic plaques, leading to rupture and—you guessed it—heart attack.

Diabetes and Heart Disease

We have long known that diabetes is a major risk factor for heart disease. A landmark clinical trial, the East-West Study, demonstrated that the risk of future heart attack in a type-2 diabetic with no prior history of coronary heart disease was similar to that of a non-diabetic *with* a prior history of a heart attack.

It is important to maintain a normal blood sugar. One way to help regulate blood sugar in your diet is by using the glycemic food index to consume less sugar overall. This is a sort of scoring system that ranks foods by how much glucose they release into the bloodstream and how quickly they do so. Each food is compared to pure glucose, which is given a score of 100.

The good news is that the best way to control blood sugar and prevent type-2 diabetes is with a healthy lifestyle. One of the key studies that highlights the importance of diet and exercise for the prevention of type-2 diabetes is the Diabetes Prevention Program (DPP). This major clinical trial separated more than three thousand overweight patients with high fasting glucose (between 100 and 125 mg/dl) into two groups. The first group, the lifestyle intervention group, received instructions regarding diet, exercise, and behavior modification. The second group took metformin, a diabetes medication designed to lower blood sugar.

THE GLYCEMIC INDEX OF A FEW COMMON FOODS

Cornflakes...81

Watermelon 72

Bagel...70

Special K cereal..69

Raisins..64

Oatmeal 58

Whole grain bread...51

Orange juice...50

Grapes 46

Apple 38

Grapefruit 25

The results of this trial were astounding: 58 percent of the patients assigned to the lifestyle intervention group reduced their risk of developing diabetes. An even more impressive 71 percent of those participants over age sixty reduced their diabetes risk. The metformin group also benefited, but not nearly as much as the lifestyle intervention group: they reduced their risk of developing diabetes by only 31 percent.

A more recent study from Spain, published in the *British Medical Journal* in May 2008, found that people who follow a Mediterranean diet are less likely to develop new-onset diabetes. Over thirteen thousand healthy men and women were enrolled in this study, which lasted more than four years. Participants who adhered most closely to a Mediterranean diet were 83 percent less likely to develop diabetes compared to those who did not follow a Mediterranean diet.

Omega-3 and Vitamin D

You will learn more about the importance of omega-3 and vitamin D for heart attack prevention in the next chapter. For now, suffice it to say that both are essential for optimal cardiovascular health. Fortunately, omega-3 and vitamin D can be measured with a blood test, and replacement therapy is advised for those who are deficient.

	High risk	Intermediate risk	Optimal
HS-Omega-3 Index (%)	< 4%	4–8%	> 8%

	High risk	Intermediate risk	Optimal
25-hydroxy-vitamin D (ng/ml)	< 15	15–29	> 30

Assignment: Get to Know Your Test Results

Now that you know what all these tests mean and why you need them, your assignment this week is to assess your own results. Compare your blood test results to the optimal values detailed in this chapter. Is your LDL cholesterol too high? Do you have too many LDL particles? Do you need to boost your HDL cholesterol levels? How much vascular inflammation do you have? Do you tend to have high blood glucose? Is your blood pressure in the optimal range?

Make sure to talk to your doctor about any abnormal lab values. The lifestyle changes you've already made will go a long way toward normalizing your results, but your doctor may also want to begin medication to get you to your goal.

For easy reference, I've included the most important test results, and their optimal results in the following chart.

The Optimal Blood Test Profile	
Lipids	
Total cholesterol	< 150 mg/dl
LDL cholesterol	< 70 mg/dl
HDL cholesterol	> 40 mg/dl (men); > 50mg/dl (women)
Non-HDL cholesterol	< 100 mg/dl
Triglycerides	< 100 mg/dl
LDL-P	< 700 nmol/L
apoB	< 60 mg/dl
LP(a) mass	< 30 mg/dl
Inflammation Biomarkers	
hs-CRP	< 1.0
Lp-PLA2	< 200
Other	
Blood pressure	< 120/80
Fasting blood sugar	< 100 mg/dl
HbA1c	< 5.7%
Hs-Omega-3-index	> 8.0%
25-hydroxy-vitamin D	> 30

WEEK FIVE

Putting It Into Practice

You're almost to the finish line! These past few weeks you've changed your diet and lifestyle, become active, and improved your stress management. Now, armed with a new understanding of what your blood test results mean and how they affect your risk of future heart attack or stroke, you can develop a plan of action with your physician to defeat cardiovascular disease—before it strikes.

This week, you should:

☐ Review your blood test results. Note the tests for which your results are suboptimal or abnormal and discuss a prevention plan involving lifestyle changes and medications (if necessary) with your physician.

☐ Look at your blood pressure. If it is not optimal, discuss ways to lower it using lifestyle changes and, if necessary, medications with your physician.

☐ Identify potential sources of chronic inflammation that may be impacting you.

☐ Create a plan to minimize sources of oxidative stress and free radical exposure from your diet and surroundings.

☐ Consciously increase the amounts of antioxidants you consume by eating a wide variety of colorful fruits and vegetables.

Heart-Healthy Supplements

C ONGRATULATIONS! You have made it to your final week of becoming Heart Attack Proof. You've made great strides over the last month and a half—stopped smoking, visited your dentist for a routine cleaning, started exercising, learned new ways to manage your stress, and tried new and delicious foods. You also had comprehensive blood tests that assessed your risk of future heart attack. You know what those blood tests mean, you know the optimal number for each, and, most importantly, you know how to improve abnormal results with lifestyle intervention and medical therapy.

In short, we've covered everything that's absolutely necessary for you to become virtually Heart Attack Proof. So this final week is devoted to something that can help strengthen your armor even further: vitamins and supplements that can be beneficial for your heart health.

Vitamins and Supplements

Vitamins are essential nutrients for optimal health that are not produced by the body in sufficient quantities and therefore must be obtained from the food we eat. Whole foods, especially a wide variety of fruits and vegetables, contain thousands of phytonutrients and antioxidants that interact with one another to help protect against things like heart disease and cancer. Mother Nature does a much better job than we can do with vitamin pills or supplements. Healthy food always trumps pills!

But just because vitamins and other supplements shouldn't be taken as a *substitute* for healthy foods doesn't mean that they don't have a place in our lives, or that they aren't beneficial at times. A daily multivitamin that contains the recommended daily allowance (RDA) for a variety of vitamins and minerals can provide an "insurance policy" against nutritional gaps in your diet. And there are other vitamins and supplements to consider for improved cardiovascular health.

Vitamin D

If there has been a recent darling of cardiovascular supplements, it is vitamin D. Researchers have identified that as much as half of North America and Western Europe may be deficient in this essential vitamin.

Our bodies produce vitamin D naturally through sun exposure. It is recommended that everyone gets about fifteen minutes of sun exposure five days a week between the hours of ten in the morning and four o'clock in the afternoon, but many of us don't. And because vitamin D is naturally found in very few foods, researchers and nutritionists are finding that supplements may be necessary.

The Institute of Medicine's 2010 RDA for vitamin D is based on age: those one to seventy years of age should get 600 IU daily, and those seventy-one years and older should get 800 IU daily.

Given the protective benefit vitamin D has shown in regards to heart disease and related cardiovascular conditions, increasing its intake could have a tremendous impact on quality of life,

VITAMIN D DAILY RECOMMENDATIONS

Age	Dose
< 70	600 IU
>70	800 IU

healthcare expenditures, and morbidity and mortality. Some of the more compelling recent data showing a link between vitamin D intake and improved cardiovascular outcomes include the following:

Researchers in Salt Lake City, Utah, found that a lack of vitamin D significantly increases risk of heart attack, stroke, and death. The study followed 27,868 people fifty years old or older for more than a year. Even in people without any previous history of heart disease, patients with very low levels of vitamin D were 77 percent more likely to die, 45 percent more likely to develop coronary artery disease, and 78 percent more likely to have a stroke compared to those with adequate levels in their blood. The findings were presented at the 2010 American Heart Association Scientific Conference in Orlando, Florida.

In a follow-up study, researchers in Utah found that those men and women who corrected their vitamin D deficiency with diet or supplements and raised their vitamin D level above 40 ng/ml had a significant reduction in their risk of heart attack and stroke.

Potassium

Potassium is an essential mineral critical for optimal heart health. Your heart's ability to beat regularly and therefore pump blood and carry oxygen to the rest of your body is dependent on electrical impulses within its muscle cells, and these impulses are regulated by electrolytes, including potassium and sodium.

When our potassium levels fall, we are more likely to develop high blood pressure and heart rhythm disorders. This is why marathon runners and those who exercise in extreme heat can have a heart rhythm disturbance and even a sudden cardiac arrest. They often become dehydrated and deplete their bodies of potassium, which can lead to a cardiac arrhythmia.

Potassium also helps the body excrete sodium, which Americans over-consume. I have seen many patients over the years who were placed on blood pressure medication, yet continued to suffer from elevated blood pressure. Simply increasing their potassium intake and decreasing the sodium in their diet could often reduce or normalize their blood pressure. The same is true for people with palpitations; often increasing the potassium stores in the body can mitigate or resolve the problem.

Most people fail to consume the recommended 4,700 mg of potassium per day, mainly because they don't eat enough fruits and vegetables, the optimal source of potassium. Foraging populations from long ago consumed, on average, five to ten times more potassium than we do today.

However, use caution when adding potassium in supplement form—never attempt to increase potassium on your own. Elevated potassium can be just as dangerous as low potassium, and people with kidney impairment or those taking potassium-sparing diuretics need to be especially careful. Your doctor can determine your potassium level and kidney function with a blood test.

Magnesium

Magnesium, like potassium, is an essential mineral that we often don't get enough of in our diets. Magnesium lowers blood pressure, stabilizes heart rhythm, and reduces the risk of heart attack and stroke. As with potassium, your doctor can check your

POTASSIUM-RICH FOODS

Try these foods that are rich in potassium to reach the recommended 4,700 mg per day. All amounts are for a serving of about 2- to 3-ounces (or 1 cup, for liquids).

Lima beans	955 mg
Wheat germ	950 mg
Soybeans (edamame)	886 mg
Spinach	839 mg
Lentils	733 mg
Carrot juice	689 mg
Apricots	544 mg
Raisins	544 mg
Avocados	540 mg
Low-fat yogurt	531 mg
Orange juice	496 mg
Bananas	467 mg
Almonds	412 mg
Non-fat milk	376 mg
Lean turkey	262 mg

magnesium level and discuss therapeutic options with you if your levels are deficient.

Coenzyme Q10

Coenzyme Q10 (CoQ10), also known as ubiquinone, is a naturally occurring antioxidant vitamin with important implications for cardiovascular health. Research is showing that CoQ10 may be beneficial for the following conditions:

- *Decreased endothelial function.* When given to patients with coronary artery disease, CoQ10 resulted in an improvement to the function of endothelial cells, cells lining the blood vessel wall that play an important role in maintaining vascular health.
- *Heart failure.* CoQ10 is important for the energy creators of our cells, the mitochondria. They are essential for heart muscle contraction. Some studies have shown an improvement in heart-pumping capacity with CoQ10, but other studies have not.
- *Angina pectoris (chest pain).* Small, preliminary studies suggest that CoQ10 may improve chest pain resulting from poor blood flow to the heart muscle.
- *Heart attack.* Preliminary study suggests that CoQ10, when given within three days of a heart attack, results in clinical benefit. Further studies are needed, however, before CoQ10 is routinely recommended in such situations.
- *Hypertension.* CoQ10 causes a small reduction in blood pressure, although its use in the treatment of hypertension remains controversial.

Statin medications, used to decrease cholesterol, can also lead to a decrease in CoQ10 levels. Since a reduction in CoQ10 may lead to muscle pain and discomfort, some physicians have advocated the use of CoQ10 supplements in all patients taking statins. However, most physicians recommend CoQ10 only if the patients develop muscle discomfort. One study revealed that 85 percent of statin users who developed muscle pain and discomfort improved following treatment with 100 mg of CoQ10 per day.

The verdict is still out on CoQ10, although it does show promise. Discuss its use with your personal physician.

Fish Oil

This is the one supplement clinically proven to benefit cardiovascular health. The omega-3 fat in fish oil is necessary for good health, and since the typical American doesn't consume enough of it from healthy food sources, sometimes relying on an omega-3 fish oil supplement is the best option.

Several large clinical trials have highlighted the value of consuming an adequate amount of fish oil, either through diet or fish oil supplements. In the US Physicians Health Study, it was shown that physicians who consumed at least one meal that included fish per week reduced their risk of sudden cardiac death by 52 percent compared to those who consumed fish only once a month. In a large Italian study, more than ten thousand men and women with preexisting heart disease were given either fish oil or a placebo. Those taking fish oil capsules had a 45 percent reduction in the risk of sudden cardiac death. In addition, a large Japanese trial of men and women with high cholesterol and high risk for heart attack found that the addition of fish oil to a statin medication resulted in a decrease in major coronary events, such as heart attack, compared to those taking the statin alone.

Whey Protein

Whey, once considered a waste by-product of cheese manufacturing, is now prized as a high-quality, protein-packed snack that is low in fat and easily digested. Whey protein has been consumed for thousands of years, yet most people are not aware of its benefits.

Especially if you want to include non-meat sources of protein in your diet, whey protein is an excellent option. Known as a "fast" protein because it's quickly absorbed into the body, whey provides a host of additional health benefits as well. Amino acids, the body's "building blocks," are necessary for the growth and repair of tissue, and whey's specific combination of these substances helps stabilize blood sugar and boosts the immune system. When it comes to heart health, whey has been found to benefit cholesterol by raising (good) HDL cholesterol and lowering triglycerides. Whey protein also promotes the growth of lean muscle and helps burn abdominal fat. In addition, research shows that whey can help manage blood glucose levels. The blood glucose levels of subjects given whey protein in combination with a pure glucose drink were significantly lower than those who only consumed the glucose drink. And like all lean proteins, whey has a thermogenic effect—it increases the basal metabolic rate, which contributes to weight control.

Regular dairy products contain lactose, which is milk sugar, but whey is lactose-free and a good choice for people who are lactose intolerant. Whey protein is generally safe; however, it too should be consumed in moderation, because excessive protein consumption can lead to kidney impairment. For most people, a whey protein smoothie or shake as a meal or snack several times a week, in addition to a healthy diet and lifestyle, is perfectly acceptable. As always, however, be sure to discuss this with your doctor.

Low-Dose Aspirin

The history of aspirin dates back thousands of years, to when the Greek physician Hippocrates used the bark and leaves of the willow tree to relieve pain and fever. The ingredient responsible for this beneficial effect was salicin—a substance that was used in 1832 to create aspirin. Soon after, aspirin was being used by physicians worldwide to treat pain, fever, and arthritis. In 1948, Dr. Lawrence Craven noted that in four hundred men to whom he prescribed aspirin, none had a heart attack, and thereafter he advised his colleagues to use daily aspirin to reduce the risk of heart attack in their patients.

We know now that aspirin works by thinning the blood—by preventing the aggregation, or clumping, of platelets, the cells that help blood to clot. Platelets contribute to clots by producing and releasing a prostaglandin called thromboxane; aspirin works because it blocks this process. Aspirin also lowers inflammation, which, as we've seen, may also contribute to a reduced risk of heart attack.

It wasn't until 1998, however, that the results of the landmark Physicians Health Study confirmed this effect. The study randomly gave more than 22,000 healthy men either aspirin or a placebo, and the study was stopped early because the results were so dramatic. There was a 44 percent decrease in the risk of a first heart attack in those men given aspirin.

Potential contraindications for aspirin use include:

- Allergy to aspirin
- Asthma
- Gastrointestinal ulcers
- History of hemorrhagic stroke
- Inherited or acquired bleeding disorders
- Reduced kidney or liver function
- Uncontrolled high blood pressure

We have evidence that aspirin is effective in women, too. In the Women's Health Study, the results of which were published in 2005 in the *New England Journal of Medicine*, aspirin reduced the incidence of stroke in women age sixty-five and older.

For those with a prior history of cardiovascular disease, such as heart attack or stroke, daily low-dose aspirin is recommended (unless there is a contraindication for its use in a particular patient).

Aspirin is not advised in patients with uncontrolled hypertension. Nevertheless, the Hypertension Optimal Treatment study in

1998 demonstrated low-dose aspirin's beneficial effect on the risk of heart attack and major cardiovascular events in patients with treated and controlled hypertension.

Most clinical studies have demonstrated that a low dose of aspirin, such as 81 mg, is as effective as larger doses of aspirin, and the risk of bleeding is lower with low-dose aspirin. Like all medications, aspirin has potential side effects, including gastrointestinal bleeding, so you should discuss the risks and benefits of regular aspirin use with your physician.

WEEK 6

Putting It Into Practice

Let's recap your journey over the last six weeks one more time:

- You've seen your personal physician and had a complete physical exam, including comprehensive blood tests.

- You had a dental evaluation and cleaning.

- You've stopped smoking.

- You've become physically active, and maybe even fit!

- Stress isn't a word that makes you, well, stressed. You're managing your stress through yoga, meditation, deep breathing, laughter, and a healthy support network.

- You are able to prepare heart-healthy meals.

- You know what your LDL particle number means and how many points you are from your optimal level.

This week, you should:

☐ Learn what vitamins and supplements are and how they can protect your heart.

☐ Learn the importance of vitamin D and omega-3 fat for heart health.

☐ Learn the benefit of low-dose aspirin for heart attack and stroke prevention.

Heart Attack Proof—At Last!

Life is not measured by the number of breaths you take,
but by every moment that takes your breath away.

—ANONYMOUS

BECOMING HEART ATTACK PROOF is rooted in living a good quality of life, choosing healthy foods that nurture your body, sharing laughter and quality time with friends and family, and taking advantage of your ability to move freely and experience life through activity and nature. It's also about optimizing your blood chemistry through a healthy lifestyle and medical therapy if necessary.

We've been using checklists to help set goals, but what you have accomplished over the last six weeks is more than just a laundry list of tasks. It is the beginning of a new way of life! The lifestyle changes you have made will not only improve your overall well-being, they will empower you to take control of your health. Cardiovascular disease is not inevitable—it *can* be defeated. Heart health, happiness, and longevity are within your grasp.

Appendices

Appendix A: Body Mass Index (BMI) Chart

Appendix B: Omega-3 (EPA and DHA) Content in Fish and Fish Oil

Appendix C: A Heart-Healthy 7-Day Meal Plan

Appendix D: The Restaurant Survival Guide

Appendix E: National Cholesterol Guidelines

Appendix F: Advanced Cardiovascular Diagnostic Tests

Appendix A

Body Mass Index (BMI) Chart

Weight in Pounds

	100	110	120	130	140	150	160	170	180	190	200	210	220	230	240	250
4'	30.5	33.6	26.6	39.7	42.7	45.8	48.8	51.9	54.9	58.0	61.0	64.1	67.1	70.2	73.2	76.3
4'2"	28.1	30.9	33.7	36.6	39.4	42.2	45.0	47.8	50.6	53.4	56.2	59.1	61.9	64.7	67.5	70.3
4'4"	26.0	28.6	31.2	33.8	36.4	39.0	41.6	44.2	46.8	49.4	52.0	54.6	57.2	59.8	62.4	65.0
4'6"	24.1	26.5	28.9	31.3	33.8	36.2	38.6	41.0	43.4	45.8	48.2	50.6	53.0	55.4	57.9	60.3
4'8"	22.4	24.7	26.9	29.1	31.4	33.6	35.9	38.1	40.4	42.6	44.8	47.1	49.3	51.6	53.8	56.0
4'10"	20.0	23.0	25.1	27.2	29.3	31.3	33.4	35.5	37.6	39.7	41.8	43.9	46.0	48.1	50.2	52.2
5'	19.5	21.5	23.4	25.4	27.3	29.3	31.2	33.2	35.2	37.1	39.1	41.0	43.0	44.9	46.9	48.8
5'2"	18.3	20.1	21.9	23.8	25.6	27.4	29.3	31.1	32.8	34.7	36.6	38.4	40.2	42.1	43.9	45.7
5'4"	17.2	18.9	20.6	22.3	24.0	25.7	27.5	29.2	30.9	32.6	34.3	36.0	37.8	39.5	41.2	42.9
5'6"	16.1	17.8	19.4	21.0	22.6	24.2	25.8	27.4	29.0	30.7	32.3	33.9	35.5	37.1	38.7	40.3
5'8"	15.2	16.7	18.2	19.8	21.3	22.8	24.3	25.8	27.4	28.9	30.4	31.9	33.4	35.0	36.5	38.0
5'10"	14.3	15.8	17.2	18.7	20.1	21.5	23.0	24.4	25.8	27.3	28.7	30.1	31.6	33.0	34.4	35.9
6'	13.6	14.9	16.3	17.6	19.0	20.3	21.7	23.1	24.4	25.8	27.1	28.5	29.8	31.2	32.5	33.9
6'2"	12.8	14.1	15.4	16.7	18.0	19.3	20.5	21.8	23.1	24.4	25.7	27.0	28.2	29.5	30.8	32.1
6'4"	12.2	13.4	14.6	15.8	17.0	18.3	19.5	20.7	21.9	23.1	24.3	25.6	26.8	28.0	29.2	30.4
6'6"	11.6	12.7	13.9	15.0	16.2	17.3	18.5	19.6	20.8	22.0	23.1	24.3	25.4	26.6	27.7	28.9
6'8"	11.0	12.1	13.2	14.3	15.4	16.5	17.6	18.7	19.8	20.9	22.0	23.1	24.2	25.3	25.4	27.5
6'10"	10.5	11.5	12.5	13.6	14.6	15.7	16.7	17.8	18.8	19.9	20.9	22.0	23.0	24.0	25.1	26.1
7'	10.0	11.0	12.0	13.0	13.9	14.9	15.9	16.9	17.9	18.9	19.9	20.9	21.9	22.9	29.9	24.9

Height in Feet and Inches

☐ Underweight   ■ Normal   ☐ Overweight   ■ Obese

Appendix B

Omega-3 (EPA and DHA) Content in Fish and Fish Oil

Fish and Seafood (per 3 oz/85 g serving)	EPA	DHA	EPA + DHA
Atlantic salmon (farmed)[2]	587	1238	1825
Pacific herring	1056	751	1807
Atlantic herring	773	939	1712
Atlantic salmon (wild)	349	1215	1564
Bluefin tuna	309	970	1279
Pink salmon (wild)	456	638	1094
Coho salmon (farmed)[2]	347	740	1087
Mackerel (canned)	369	677	1046
Sockeye salmon (wild)	451	595	1046
Chum salmon (canned)	402	597	999
Rainbow trout (farmed)[2]	284	697	981
Coho salmon (wild)	341	559	900
Sardines (canned)	402	433	835
Albacore/white tuna (canned)[3]	198	535	733
Shark (raw)	267	444	711
Swordfish[3]	117	579	696
Sea bass	175	473	648
Pollock	77	383	460
Flat fish (flounder/sole)	207	219	426

Fish and Seafood (per 3 oz/85 g serving)	EPA	DHA	EPA + DHA
Blue crab	207	196	403
Halibut	77	318	395
Oysters (farmed)[2]	195	179	374
King crab	251	100	351
Walleye	93	245	338
Dungeness crab	239	96	335
Scallops	141	169	310
Skipjack tuna	77	201	278
Shrimp	145	122	267
Clams	117	124	241
Yellowfin tuna	40	197	237
Light chunk tuna	40	190	230
Catfish (wild)	85	116	201
Catfish (farmed)[2]	42	109	151
Cod	3	131	134
Mahi-mahi (dolphin fish)	22	96	118
Tilapia	4	111	115
Orange roughy	5	21	26
Dietary Supplements (per 1,000 mg capsule, or 1 tsp)			
Standard drug store fish oil capsules	180	120	300
Fish oil concentrates (many varieties)	100–400	100–400	300–700
Cod liver oil (teaspoon)	300	500	800

Table provided by Health Diagnostic Laboratory and adapted from Harris et al., Current Atherosclerosis Reports 2008; 10: 503–509.

[1] Based on USDA Nutrient Data Lab values. Values are for fish cooked with dry heat, unless otherwise noted.

[2] Although there has been some concern regarding the presence of small amounts of environmental pollutants in some types of farmed fish, the overall health benefit from the omega-3s present in these fish has been determined to far outweigh the risks (*Journal of the American Medical Association* 2006; 296: 1885–1899).

[3] Because of the possibility for mercury contamination, the FDA and EPA recommend that these fish (along with king mackerel and tilefish) not be consumed by women who are already or are trying to become pregnant, nursing mothers, and children under the age of two. For all other people, the intake of these fish should be limited to 6 oz per week (or 12 oz per week for albacore tuna).
HS-Omega-3 Index® and OmegaQuant® are registered marks of Harris Scientific, Inc. and used with written permission.

The benefits and risks of eating fish vary depending on a person's stage of life:

- Children and pregnant women are advised by the U.S. Food and Drug Administration to avoid eating those fish with the potential for the highest level of mercury contamination (e.g., shark, swordfish, king mackerel, or tilefish).
- For middle-aged and older men and women, the benefits of fish consumption far outweigh the potential risks.

Eating a variety of fish will help minimize any potentially adverse effects due to environmental pollutants. Potential exposure to some contaminants can be reduced by removing the skin and surface fat from fish before cooking.

Appendix C

A Heart-Healthy
7-Day Meal Plan

This sample 7-day meal plan, drawn from my book *The Miami Mediterranean Diet*, will help you get started on your way to losing weight and lowering your risk of heart disease.

For more information, including over three hundred heart-healthy recipes, pick up a copy of *The Miami Mediterranean Diet*.

DAY 1

BREAKFAST

    4 ounces vegetable or fruit juice

    1 slice whole wheat toast with extra-virgin olive oil or 1 teaspoon vegetable spread (trans fat–free canola/olive oil spread)

    1 teaspoon jam

    ½ cup plain low-fat yogurt (sweetened with non-caloric sweetener if desired)

    ½ cup blueberries or strawberries

    8 ounces water

    Coffee or tea (soy or non-fat milk, trans fat–free coffee creamer, and noncaloric sweetener if desired)

APPROX. 239 CALORIES

OPTIONAL MIDMORNING SNACK

10–20 almonds or walnuts
8 ounces water or non-caloric beverage

LUNCH

Chickpea Pita Pocket (page 182)
1 medium apple, sliced and drizzled with honey
8 ounces water or non-caloric beverage

APPROX. 319 CALORIES

OPTIONAL MIDDAY SNACK

10–20 almonds or walnuts
8 ounces water or non-caloric beverage

DINNER

1 jumbo clove Roasted Garlic (page 171)
½ (6-inch) whole wheat pita loaf, split open, sprayed with olive oil and
  herb seasonings of choice, and toasted in the microwave or oven until
  crispy
Goat Cheese Stuffed Tomato (page 171)
Linguine and Mixed Seafood (page 184)
Fresh vegetable of choice (flavor with olive oil or vegetable spread as desired)
Drunken Apricots (page 192)
8 ounces water
1 or 2 (4-ounce) glasses of red wine or purple grape juice
Coffee or tea (soy milk or non-fat, trans fat–free coffee creamer and
  noncaloric sweetener if desired)

APPROX. 761 CALORIES

OPTIONAL EVENING SNACK

1 apple or orange
8 ounces water

DAY 2

BREAKFAST

4 ounces vegetable or fruit juice

½ cup egg whites with diced onions, tomato, and green bell peppers cooked into an omelet

1 slice whole wheat toast with extra-virgin olive oil or 1 teaspoon vegetable spread (trans fat–free canola/olive oil spread)

1 teaspoon fruit jam

½ small banana

8 ounces water

Coffee or tea (soy or non-fat milk, trans fat–free coffee creamer, and noncaloric sweetener if desired)

APPROX. 230 CALORIES

OPTIONAL MIDMORNING SNACK

10–20 almonds or walnuts

8 ounces water or non-caloric beverage

LUNCH

Greek Olive and Feta Cheese Pasta Salad (page 172)

½ (6-inch) whole wheat pita loaf, toasted if desired

⅛-inch fresh cantaloupe

8 ounces water or non-caloric beverage

APPROX. 354 CALORIES

OPTIONAL MIDDAY SNACK

1 apple

8 ounces water or non-caloric beverage

DINNER

1 jumbo clove Roasted Garlic (page 171)

½ (6-inch) whole wheat pita loaf, split open, sprayed with olive oil and herb seasonings of choice, and toasted until crispy in the oven or microwave

6–8 marinated assorted olives
Grilled Citrus Salmon with Garlic Greens (page 185)
Grilled Eggplant (page 190)
Strawberries and Balsamic Syrup (page 193)
8 ounces water
1 or 2 (4-ounce) glasses of red wine or purple grape juice
Coffee or tea (soy or non-fat milk, trans fat–free coffee creamer, and
    noncaloric sweetener if desired)

APPROX. 653 CALORIES

OPTIONAL EVENING SNACK
1 apple or orange
8 ounces water

DAY 3

BREAKFAST
4 ounces vegetable or fruit juice
½ cup egg whites with diced onions, tomato, and green bell peppers
1 slice whole wheat toast with olive oil (extra-virgin) or 1 teaspoon veg-
    etable spread (trans fat–free canola/olive oil spread)
1 teaspoon fruit jam
1 medium fresh peach or 1 large plum
8 ounces water
Coffee or tea (soy or non-fat milk, trans fat–free coffee creamer, and
    noncaloric sweetener if desired)

APPROX. 230 CALORIES

OPTIONAL MIDMORNING SNACK
10–20 almonds or walnuts
8 ounces water or non-caloric beverage
Lunch
Italian Minestrone Soup with Pesto (page 177)
1 slice whole grain crusty bread with extra-virgin olive oil

½ cup fresh raspberries

½ cup plain low-fat yogurt, sweetened with non-caloric sweetener if
desired

8 ounces water or non-caloric beverage

APPROX. 390 CALORIES

OPTIONAL MIDDAY SNACK

1 apple

8 ounces water or non-caloric beverage

DINNER

Simple Spanish Salad (page 173)

1 jumbo clove Roasted Garlic (page 171)

½ (6-inch) whole wheat pita loaf, split open, sprayed with olive oil and
herb seasonings of choice, and toasted until crispy in the oven or
microwave

1 slice soft goat cheese

6–8 marinated mixed olives

Fresh vegetable of choice (flavor with olive oil or vegetable spread as
desired)

Chicken Piccata (page 186)

Honeydew Sorbet (page 194)

8 ounces water

1 or 2 (4-ounce) glasses of red wine or purple grape juice

Coffee or tea (soy or non-fat milk, trans fat–free coffee creamer, and
noncaloric sweetener if desired)

APPROX. 725 CALORIES

OPTIONAL EVENING SNACK

2 Meringue Cookies (page 194)

Green tea or 8 ounces water

DAY 4

BREAKFAST

4 ounces vegetable or fruit juice
2 slices whole wheat toast
2 tablespoons fresh chunky peanut butter
2 teaspoons honey
½ ruby red grapefruit, sweetened with non-caloric sweetener if desired
8 ounces water
Coffee or tea (soy or non-fat milk, trans fat–free coffee creamer, and noncaloric sweetener if desired)

APPROX. 385 CALORIES

OPTIONAL MIDMORNING SNACK

10–20 almonds or walnuts
8 ounces water or non-caloric beverage

LUNCH

Light Caesar Salad (page 174)
1 slice Margherita Pizza (page 181)
10–20 seedless grapes
8 ounces water or non-caloric beverage

APPROX. 302 CALORIES

OPTIONAL MIDDAY SNACK

1 apple
8 ounces water or non-caloric beverage

DINNER

1 clove jumbo Roasted Garlic (page 171)
½ (6-inch) whole wheat pita loaf, split open, sprayed with extra-virgin olive oil and herb seasonings of choice, and toasted until crispy in the oven or microwave
Chilly Tomato Soup (page 178)

Fennel Salad (page 174)

Fresh vegetable of choice (flavor with olive oil or vegetable spread as desired)

Spicy Whole Wheat Capellini with Garlic (page 187)

8 ounces water

Sweet Plum Compote (page 195)

1 or 2 (4-ounce) glasses of red wine or purple grape juice

Coffee or tea (soy or non-fat milk, trans fat–free coffee creamer, and noncaloric sweetener if desired)

APPROX. 786 CALORIES

OPTIONAL EVENING SNACK

1 apple or orange

8 ounces water

DAY 5

BREAKFAST

4 ounces vegetable or fruit juice

1 slice whole wheat toast with extra-virgin olive oil or 1 teaspoon vegetable spread (trans fat–free canola/olive oil spread)

1 teaspoon fruit jam

½ cup plain low-fat yogurt, sweetened with non-caloric sweetener if desired

½ cup blueberries or strawberries

8 ounces water

Coffee or tea (soy or non-fat milk, trans fat–free coffee creamer, and noncaloric sweetener if desired)

APPROX. 289 CALORIES

OPTIONAL MIDMORNING SNACK

10–20 almonds or walnuts

8 ounces water or non-caloric beverage

LUNCH

Hearty Bean Soup (page 179)
1 slice whole grain bread with extra-virgin olive oil or 1 teaspoon veg-
etable spread (trans fat–free canola/olive oil spread)
3 fresh apricots
8 ounces water or non-caloric beverage

APPROX. 414 CALORIES

OPTIONAL MIDDAY SNACK

1 apple
8 ounces water or non-caloric beverage

DINNER

4 tablespoons hummus
½ (6-inch) whole wheat pita loaf, split open, sprayed with extra-virgin
olive oil and herb seasonings of choice, and toasted until crispy in the
oven or microwave
4 tomato wedges topped with slivers of red onion, freshly grated mozza-
rella cheese, chopped fresh cilantro, and drizzled with aged balsamic
vinegar and 1 teaspoon extra-virgin olive oil.
Fettuccine with Smoked Salmon and Basil Pesto (page 188)
Peach Marsala Compote (page 196)
1 or 2 (4-ounce) glasses of red wine or purple grape juice
8 ounces water
Coffee or tea (soy or non-fat milk, trans fat–free coffee creamer, and
noncaloric sweetener if desired)

APPROX. 774 CALORIES

OPTIONAL EVENING SNACK

2 Meringue Cookies (page 194)
Green tea or 8 ounces water

DAY 6

BREAKFAST

4 ounces vegetable or fruit juice
½ cup dry oatmeal, cooked and sweetened with non-caloric sweetener if
desired
1 tablespoon seedless black raisins
1 medium orange, sliced
8 ounces water
Coffee or tea (soy or non-fat milk, trans fat–free coffee creamer, and
noncaloric sweetener if desired)

APPROX. 292 CALORIES

OPTIONAL MIDMORNING SNACK

10–20 almonds or walnuts
8 ounces water or non-caloric beverage

LUNCH

Veggie Wrap (page 183)
Roasted Peppers (page 191)
6–8 marinated mixed olives
1 medium fresh pear, peach, or apple
8 ounces water or non-caloric beverage

APPROX. 601 CALORIES

OPTIONAL MIDDAY SNACK

1 apple
8 ounces water or non-caloric beverage

DINNER

1 jumbo clove Roasted Garlic (page 171)
½ (6-inch) whole wheat pita loaf, split open, sprayed with olive oil and
herb seasonings, and toasted until crispy in the oven or microwave
Mediterranean Mixed Greens (page 175)

Baked Tilapia (page 188)
Classic Spinach and Pine Nuts (page 176)
Strawberries Amaretto (page 196)
8 ounces water
1 or 2 (4-ounce) glasses of red wine or purple grape juice coffee or tea
  (soy or non-fat milk, trans fat–free coffee creamer, and non-caloric
  sweetener if desired)

APPROX. 597 CALORIES

OPTIONAL EVENING SNACK
2 Meringue Cookies (page 194)
Green tea or 8 ounces water

DAY 7

BREAKFAST
4 ounces vegetable or fruit juice
½ cup egg whites with diced red onion, tomato, and green bell peppers
  cooked into an omelet
1 slice whole wheat toast with extra-virgin olive oil or 1 teaspoon veg-
  etable spread (trans fat–free canola/olive oil spread)
1 teaspoon fruit jam
1 purple plum
8 ounces water
Coffee or tea (soy or non-fat milk, trans fat–free coffee creamer, and
  noncaloric sweetener if desired)

APPROX. 230 CALORIES

OPTIONAL MIDMORNING SNACK
10–20 almonds or walnuts
8 ounces water or non-caloric beverage

LUNCH

Eggplant Soup (page 180)
1 slice whole grain crusty bread, drizzled with extra-virgin olive oil and
herb seasonings of choice
1 large kiwi fruit, sliced
½ cup fresh strawberries, sliced
8 ounces water or non-caloric beverage

APPROX. 420 CALORIES

OPTIONAL MIDDAY SNACK

1 apple
8 ounces water or non-caloric beverage

DINNER

1 slice whole grain bread with extra-virgin olive oil and herb seasonings
of choice
6–8 marinated assorted olives
Broccoli with Fresh Garlic (page 192)
Fettuccine with Sundried Tomatoes and Goat Cheese (page 189)
Fresh Fruit Kebobs and Cinnamon Honey Dip (page 197)
8 ounces water
1 or 2 (4-ounce) glasses of red wine or purple grape juice
Coffee or tea (soy or non-fat milk, trans fat–free coffee creamer, and
noncaloric sweetener if desired)

APPROX. 1050 CALORIES

OPTIONAL EVENING SNACK

1 apple or orange
8 ounces water

Recipes

APPETIZERS

Roasted Garlic
(MAKES 4–5 SERVINGS)

1 elephant jumbo garlic head
Extra-virgin olive oil to drizzle
Dry seasonings of choice (optional)

Holding entire head of garlic, cut off the top leaf points of each clove to expose a small portion of the clove. Keep the remainder of leaves intact around the body of the garlic head. Place trimmed garlic head in a tight-fitting oven-safe bowl, trimmed side up. Drizzle a small amount of olive oil over the top of the head and down around the sides. Sprinkle with your favorite seasoning (optional). Place garlic on middle rack of oven and bake at 400 degrees for 20–30 minutes, or until cloves are soft and a light golden brown. Remove from oven and spread garlic on crusty bread, or add to vegetables, omelets, or pasta.

Approx. 59 calories per serving
3g protein, 0.2g total fat, <1g saturated fat, 0 trans fat,
13g carbohydrates, 0 cholesterol, 7mg sodium, 1g fiber

Goat Cheese Stuffed Tomatoes
(MAKES 2 SERVINGS)

6–8 leaves arugula
2 medium ripe tomatoes
3 ounces crumbled goat cheese
Salt and pepper to taste
Balsamic vinegar

Extra-virgin olive oil
Red onion, very thinly sliced
Fresh chopped parsley

Place 3–4 leaves arugula in the center of each salad plate. Cut tops
(about ¼ inch) off the tomatoes. With a paring knife, core out the center of the tomatoes, about ½ inch deep. Fill tomatoes with crumbled feta
cheese, add salt and pepper to taste, and drizzle with balsamic vinegar
and extra-virgin olive oil. Garnish with red onion slices and chopped
parsley. Serve at room temperature.

Approx. 142 calories per serving
7g protein, 13g total fat, 3g saturated fat, 0 trans fat, 7g carbohydrates,
37mg cholesterol, 485mg sodium, 1g fiber

SALADS

Greek Olive and Feta Cheese Pasta
(MAKES 4 SERVINGS)

4 ½ ounces ziti pasta
3 ounces crumbled feta cheese
10 small Greek olives, pitted and coarsely chopped
¼ cup fresh, coarsely chopped basil leaves
2 cloves garlic, finely minced
1 tablespoon extra-virgin olive oil
¼ teaspoon finely chopped hot pepper
½ red bell pepper, diced
½ yellow bell pepper, diced
2 plum tomatoes, seeded and diced

Bring water to a boil, add pasta, and cook pasta until al dente. Remove
from heat, drain pasta, and return to pot, drizzling with scant amount

of olive oil to keep pasta from sticking together. Set aside. In a large serving bowl combine feta cheese, olives, basil, garlic, olive oil, and hot peppers then set aside for 30 minutes. Add cooked pasta, red and yellow bell peppers, and tomato; toss ingredients well. Cover and refrigerate for at least 1 hour, until well chilled. Toss again before serving. This salad goes well as a side dish to grilled lamb or fish.

Approx. 235 calories per serving
7g protein, 10g total fat, 1g saturated fat, 0 trans fat,
27g carbohydrates, 18mg cholesterol, 98mg sodium, 2g fiber

Simple Spanish Salad
(MAKES 6 SERVINGS)

1 bag (2 bunches) cleaned and trimmed romaine lettuce, torn into bite-sized pieces
3 medium ripe tomatoes cut into ¼-inch wedges
1 large sweet onion, thinly sliced
1 green bell pepper, seeded and thinly sliced
1 red bell pepper, seeded and thinly sliced
¼ cup chopped and pitted marinated green olives
¼ cup chopped and pitted black olives
¼ cup extra-virgin olive oil
3 tablespoons balsamic vinegar
Salt and freshly ground pepper to taste

Place a bed of romaine lettuce on six chilled salad plates. Arrange tomatoes, onions, peppers, and olives on top of the lettuce on each plate. Mix olive oil and vinegar together; drizzle over salad. Add salt and pepper if desired and serve.

Approx. 107 calories per serving
2g protein, 9g total fat, 1g saturated fat, 0 trans fat,
7g carbohydrates, 0 cholesterol, 145mg sodium, 3g fiber

Light Caesar Salad
(MAKES 6 SERVINGS)

1–2 bunches packaged pre-cleaned romaine lettuce, torn in pieces
½ cup non-fat plain yogurt
2 teaspoons lemon juice
2 ½ teaspoons balsamic vinegar
1 teaspoon Worcestershire sauce
2 cloves freshly minced garlic
½ teaspoon anchovy paste
½ cup grated Parmesan cheese
10 small pitted black olives, chopped

Clean and pat dry romaine lettuce and place in large salad bowl. In a blender mix yogurt, lemon juice, vinegar, Worcestershire sauce, garlic, anchovy paste, and ¼ cup Parmesan cheese until smooth. Pour mixture over lettuce and toss. Garnish with remaining cheese and olives.

Approx. 49 calories per serving
4g protein, 1g total fat, <0.1g saturated fat, 0 trans fat,
4g carbohydrates, 4mg cholesterol, 112mg sodium, 1g fiber

Fennel Salad
(MAKES 4–6 SERVINGS)

1 large clove garlic, halved
1 large fennel bulb, thinly sliced
½ English cucumber, thinly sliced
1 tablespoon minced fresh chives
8 large radishes, thinly sliced
3 tablespoons extra-virgin olive oil
2 ½ tablespoons freshly squeezed lemon juice
Salt and freshly ground pepper to taste
Marinated mixed olives (optional)

Rub the inside of a large bowl with garlic. Add fennel, cucumber, chives, and radishes. In a separate bowl whisk together olive oil, fresh lemon juice, and salt and pepper to taste. Pour olive oil mixture over salad and toss to mix. Garnish with marinated olives if desired.

Approx. 76 calories per serving
0 protein, 10g total fat, 1g saturated fat, 0 trans fat,
3g carbohydrates, 2mg cholesterol, 20mg sodium, 1g fiber

Mediterranean Mixed Greens
(MAKES 4–6 SERVINGS)

6 cups assorted fresh mixed greens (such as arugula, radicchio, baby
    spinach, watercress, and romaine)
1 small red onion, thinly sliced and separated into rings
20 firm cherry tomatoes, halved
¼ cup chopped walnuts
¼ cup dried cranberries

FOR DRESSING:
2 tablespoons balsamic vinegar
4 tablespoons extra-virgin olive oil
1 tablespoon water
½ teaspoon crushed dried oregano
2 cloves garlic, finely minced
Crumbled feta cheese (optional)
Coarsely ground fresh pepper to taste

In a large salad bowl, combine greens, onion, tomatoes, walnuts, and cranberries. Gently toss.

DRESSING: Combine vinegar, oil, water, oregano, and garlic; shake well. Pour dressing over salad and toss lightly to coat. Garnish with feta cheese, if desired, and fresh pepper.

Approx. 140 calories per serving
2g protein, 12g total fat, 1g saturated fat, 0 trans fat,
6g carbohydrates, 0 cholesterol, 47mg sodium, 1g fiber

Classic Spinach And Pine Nuts
(MAKES 4 SERVINGS)

¼ cup golden raisins
4 tablespoons pine nuts
2 tablespoons extra-virgin olive oil
4 cloves garlic, chopped
1½ (10-ounce) bags fresh spinach, cleaned
Salt and freshly ground pepper to taste
Fresh lemon juice
Extra-virgin olive oil to taste

Place raisins in a bowl and cover with boiling water. Let stand for approximately 10 minutes, until raisins are plump; drain well. In a skillet over medium heat, toast pine nuts, stirring constantly for about 1–2 minutes. Remove from heat, and set aside. In a large skillet, warm olive oil. Add garlic and sauté for 1–2 minutes, until golden. Add spinach a little at a time until it all becomes wilted (about 3–5 minutes), stirring constantly. Pour raisins over spinach and mix well. With a slotted spoon, transfer spinach to a serving dish, and sprinkle pine nuts over top. Serve immediately or, if serving at room temperature, add fresh lemon juice and extra-virgin olive oil to taste.

Approx. 149 calories per serving
4g protein, 12g total fat, 2g saturated fat, 0 trans fat,
10g carbohydrates, 0 cholesterol, 41mg sodium, 2g fiber

SOUPS

Italian Minestrone Soup with Pesto
(MAKES 6–8 SERVINGS)

1 cup dried cannellini beans
4 cups low-sodium, fat-free chicken broth
4 cups water
2 medium white potatoes, peeled and diced
2 ounces dry ditalini pasta
2 large carrots, chopped
3 stalks celery, chopped
½ cup chopped white onion
2 cloves garlic, minced
1 cup tomato juice
3 plum tomatoes, chopped
1 large zucchini, chopped
Freshly shredded Parmesan cheese for garnish (optional)
For pesto:
1 cup fresh basil leaves
1 teaspoon crumbled dried basil leaves
4 cloves garlic, finely minced
3 tablespoons extra-virgin olive oil
½ cup grated Parmesan cheese
Salt and freshly ground pepper to taste

Rinse dried cannellini beans and place in a large covered pot. Add chicken broth and water and bring to a boil. Uncover pot, reduce heat and simmer until beans are tender; roughly 1 hour. Add potatoes, pasta, carrots, celery, onion, garlic, and tomato juice. Return mixture to a boil, then reduce heat and simmer uncovered for 10 minutes. Add tomatoes and zucchini, and simmer until all are tender. Process pesto ingredients in a food processor or blender until finely chopped. Remove soup from heat and stir in pesto mixture, and serve garnished with Parmesan cheese if desired.

Approx. 182 calories per serving without pesto
10g protein, 1g total fat, 0 saturated fat, 0 trans fat,
20g carbohydrates, 3mg cholesterol, 204mg sodium, 4g fiber

Approx. 254 calories per serving with pesto added
12g protein, 8g total fat, 2g saturated fat, 0 trans fat,
20g carbohydrates, 10mg cholesterol, 291mg sodium, 4g fiber

Chilly Tomato Soup
(MAKES 4 SERVINGS)

10 medium ripe tomatoes
½ tablespoon extra-virgin olive oil
4–5 cloves garlic, minced
2 tablespoons chopped onions
2 cups low-sodium, fat-free chicken broth
2 teaspoons low-calorie baking sweetener
½ teaspoon fresh basil, chopped
Salt and freshly ground pepper to taste
8 scallions, chopped (optional)
2 cucumbers, diced (optional)
1 large green zucchini, diced (optional)

In a large pot of boiling water, dip tomatoes for 30 seconds, then immediately place tomatoes in cold water. Allow to sit until they can be handled. Skin tomatoes with a paring knife, cut in half crosswise, and remove seeds. Core and then cut into quarter pieces. In a blender or food processor, process tomatoes until pureed. In a skillet, heat olive oil and sauté garlic and onions until tender. Remove from heat. In a large bowl, combine pureed tomatoes, sautéed onion mixture, chicken broth, sweetener, basil, and salt and pepper, stirring to mix ingredients together. Refrigerate soup for 4–6 hours until well chilled. Garnish with scallions, cucumbers, and zucchini if desired.

Approx. 161 calories per serving

10g protein, <0.5g total fat, 0 saturated fat, 0 trans fat,
65g carbohydrates, 5mg cholesterol, 197mg sodium, 1g fiber

Hearty Bean Soup
(MAKES 6–8 SERVINGS)

2 cups water
2 medium potatoes, peeled and coarsely chopped
2 large carrots, coarsely chopped
2 stalks celery, coarsely chopped
1 bay leaf
1 tablespoon fresh thyme
Salt and freshly ground pepper to taste
3 tablespoons extra-virgin olive oil
5 cloves fresh garlic, minced
1 medium onion, finely chopped
½ small hot pepper, finely chopped
5 cups low-sodium, fat-free chicken broth
4 (15-ounce) cans Great Northern beans
Salt and freshly ground pepper to taste
Grated Parmesan cheese (optional)
Chopped fresh flat leaf parsley (optional)

In a heavy pot, combine water, potato, carrots, celery, bay leaf, thyme, and salt and pepper. Bring to a boil, reduce heat, cover, and simmer until vegetables are tender. While vegetables are cooking, combine oil, garlic, onion, and hot pepper in a large skillet, and sauté until tender and lightly browned. Add 1 cup of chicken broth and beans to garlic mixture, mix together well, cover, and simmer for about 10 minutes to allow flavors to blend. Add salt and pepper to taste. Combine bean mixture and 4 cups of chicken broth, and add to vegetable pot. Stir to mix, then keep at a low simmer for about 10–15 minutes, allowing flavors to blend. Garnish with cheese and parsley, if desired.

Approx. 220 calories per serving

11g protein, 6g total fat, 0.7g saturated fat, 0 trans fat,
36g carbohydrates, 3mg cholesterol, 663mg sodium, 9g fiber

Eggplant Soup
(MAKES 4–6 SERVINGS)

2 tablespoons extra-virgin olive oil
2 cloves fresh garlic, minced
½ medium onion, thinly sliced and separated into rings
1 medium eggplant, peeled and cut into ½-inch cubes
½ teaspoon oregano
¼ teaspoon thyme
4 cups low-sodium, fat-free chicken broth
½ cup dry sherry
Salt and freshly ground pepper to taste
1 large tomato, sliced
10 ounces non-fat feta cheese, crumbled
Freshly grated Parmesan cheese (optional)

Heat oil in large skillet over medium heat; add garlic and onion, and
sauté until lightly golden. Add eggplant, oregano, and thyme; continue
cooking until eggplant browns slightly, stirring constantly. Reduce heat
to low, add broth, cover, and simmer for roughly 5 minutes. Add sherry,
cover, and continue to simmer for another 2–3 minutes. Stir in salt and
pepper to taste if needed, and remove from heat. Allow to cool slightly.
Preheat broiler, and pour slightly cooled soup into an oven-safe bowl.
Top soup with tomato slices and feta cheese, place soup under broiler,
and heat until feta melts into soup. Garnish with grated Parmesan
cheese if desired, and broil until cheese is browned.

Approx. 146 calories per serving
9g protein, 5g total fat, <1g saturated fat, 0 trans fat,
10g carbohydrates, 3mg cholesterol, 538mg sodium, 2g fiber

PIZZA

Pizza Margherita
(MAKES AN 8-SLICE, 15-INCH PIZZA)

Thin Crust Pizza Dough (page 181)
4 Roma tomatoes, thinly sliced
Salt and freshly ground pepper to taste
½ cup yellow sweet pepper, thinly sliced
¾ cup shredded part-skim mozzarella cheese, about 3 ounces
4–5 snipped fresh basil leaves
¼ cup freshly grated Parmesan cheese
1 tablespoon extra-virgin olive oil

Preheat oven to 450 degrees. Follow directions for pizza dough and roll out to a 12–15-inch round. Place dough on a scantly oiled pizza pan. Spread tomatoes on rolled-out dough almost to the edge of the crust. Sprinkle with salt and pepper to taste. Top tomatoes with yellow peppers, mozzarella cheese, basil, and Parmesan cheese, and drizzle olive oil over the top. Bake at 450 degrees for 8–10 minutes or until crust is crisp and cheeses are melted.

Approx. 202 calories per slice
11g protein, 7g total fat, 3g saturated fat, 0 trans fat,
28g carbohydrates, 7mg cholesterol, 375mg sodium, 1g fiber

Thin Crust Pizza Dough
(MAKES AN 8-SLICE, 15-INCH CRUST)

1⅔ cups unbleached all-purpose flour
½ teaspoon salt
1 package dry active yeast
2 tablespoons extra-virgin olive oil
½ cup warm water
Olive oil to lightly coat pan

Put flour, salt, and yeast in a large bowl and mix with a wooden spoon. Make a well in the center and add oil and water. Gradually work in flour from the sides of the brown as the mixture becomes smooth, pliable, soft dough. If too sticky, sprinkle a little more flour into the mixture, but don't make the dough dry. Transfer dough to a lightly floured surface and knead for about 10 minutes; add very small amounts of flour if needed until dough becomes smooth and elastic. Rub a small amount of oil over the surface of the dough, then return it to a clean bowl, cover it with a cloth, and place it in a warm area for about 1 hour or until dough doubles in size. Remove dough to a lightly floured surface, knead for an additional 2 minutes, then roll out into a 15-inch round. Place on pizza pan and top with sauce and ingredients of choice. Bake at 425 degrees until crust is crispy.

Approx. 115 calories per slice, crust only
2g protein, 3g total fat, <0.5g saturated fat, 0 trans fat,
18 carbohydrates, 0 cholesterol, 144mg sodium, 0 fiber

WRAPS AND SANDWICHES

Chickpea Pita Pockets
(MAKES 8 SERVINGS)

1 (15-ounce) can chickpeas, rinsed and drained
1 cup shredded fresh spinach
⅔ cup halved seedless red grapes
½ cup finely chopped red bell pepper
⅓ cup thinly sliced celery
½ medium cucumber, diced
¼ cup finely chopped onion
¼ cup light mayonnaise
1 tablespoon balsamic syrup
½ tablespoon poppy seed
4 (6-inch) whole wheat pita loaves, cut in half

In a large bowl combine chickpeas, spinach, grapes, red pepper, celery, cucumber, and onion. Whisk together mayonnaise, balsamic syrup, and poppy seeds. Add poppy seed mixture to chickpea mixture, and stir until well blended. Lightly toast pita halves and fill with chickpea filling. Serve.

Approx. 152 calories per serving
7g protein, 3g total fat, 0.3g saturated fat, 0 trans fat,
29g carbohydrates, 3mg cholesterol, 294mg sodium, 5g fiber

Veggie Wrap
(MAKES 6 SERVINGS)

Olive oil cooking spray
2 medium tomatoes, cut into ½-inch thick slices
2 small cucumbers, sliced lengthwise into ½-inch thick slices
2 small onions, cut into ½-inch thick slices
1 green bell pepper, cut into strips
2 medium zucchini, sliced lengthwise into ½-inch thick slices
Extra-virgin olive oil to drizzle
¾ tablespoon crumbled dried oregano
¼ tablespoon crumbled dried rosemary
¾ teaspoon dried thyme
½ (7-ounce) can chickpeas, rinsed and drained
¼ teaspoon cumin (optional)
Salt and freshly ground pepper to taste
Alfalfa sprouts (optional)
6 whole wheat flat bread (8–10-inch), warmed

Spray non-stick pan with cooking spray. Place tomatoes, cucumbers, onions, peppers, and zucchini on pan, and drizzle with olive oil. Sprinkle with oregano, rosemary, and thyme, and roast for 15–20 minutes at 425 degrees. Add chickpeas and cumin, plus salt and pepper to taste, and cook an additional 15–20 minutes until tender. Fill warmed flat bread with bean and veggie mix, top with alfalfa sprouts, roll up, and serve.

Approx. 170 calories per serving
8g protein, 1g total fat, <0.3g saturated fat, 0 trans fat
36g carbohydrates, 0 cholesterol, 325mg sodium, 6g fiber

MAIN DISHES

Linguine and Mixed Seafood

(MAKES 4–6 SERVINGS)

8 ounces natural clam juice
2 cups good dry wine (not cooking wine)
¼ pound baby octopus, cleaned
¼ pound shrimp, peeled and deveined
¼ pound calamari, cleaned, cut into ¼-inch rings
20 mussels, scrubbed and debearded (discard any open mussels)
¼ pound bay scallops
3 tablespoons extra-virgin olive oil
3–4 cloves garlic , minced
¼ teaspoon freshly chopped hot peppers
8 small ripe plum tomatoes, chopped into small chunks
Pinch of low-calorie baking sweetener
½ tablespoon chopped fresh parsley
½ tablespoon chopped fresh oregano
Salt and freshly ground pepper to taste
½ pound linguine
10–12 arugula leaves, chopped
10 pitted Kalamata black olives, halved

In a large deep skillet, add clam juice, wine, octopus, shrimp, calamari, mussels, and scallops. Bring to boil, cover, and reduce heat to simmer, stirring occasionally, until calamari and octopus are almost tender. Remove mussels and shell all but 9–12; set these aside for garnish and return shelled mussels to seafood skillet to keep warm. In a separate skillet, over medium heat, add oil and garlic, and sauté until golden brown. Add hot peppers to garlic mixture, reduce heat to simmer, and cook for 1–2 additional minutes. Add tomatoes, sweetener, parsley, oregano, and salt and pepper to taste, and simmer another 3–4 minutes. Cover to keep warm, and set aside. Bring water to a boil, add pasta, and cook pasta until al dente. Remove from heat, drain pasta, and return to pot, drizzling with scant amount of olive oil to keep pasta from sticking together. Set aside. With a slotted spoon remove seafood from skillet and strain remaining liquid through sieve or cheesecloth. Return seafood and 1 cup of strained liquid to skillet; add pasta and tomato mixture, and toss all ingredients. Spoon entire linguini and seafood dish into a large pasta bowl, garnish with chopped arugula, black olives, and remaining unshelled mussels, and serve.

Approx. 375 calories per serving
21g protein, 8g total fat, 1g saturated fat, 0 trans fat,
34g carbohydrates, 98mg cholesterol, 235mg sodium, 2g fiber

Grilled Citrus Salmon with Garlic Greens
(MAKES 4 SERVINGS)

¼ cup orange marmalade
2 tablespoons fresh lime juice
2 tablespoons fresh lemon juice
¼ cup low-sodium soy sauce
3 teaspoons grated orange rind
4 (3-ounce) salmon fillets
2 teaspoons extra-virgin olive oil
2 teaspoons minced garlic
2 (10-ounce) bags fresh spinach
Scant amount of olive oil to rub on fish
Salt and pepper to taste
1 teaspoon fresh garlic, mashed to rub on fish
1 heaping tablespoon capers, drained
1 tablespoon balsamic vinegar
4 scallions, white and light green parts, thinly sliced (2–3 inch lengths)

Whisk together marmalade, lime and lemon juices, soy sauce, and orange rind; pour mixture over fillets and marinade for 30 minutes in refrigerator. Prepare grill or preheat broiler. Heat olive oil in a heavy skillet over medium-high heat; add garlic and spinach, one bag at a time, and sauté, stirring often, until spinach is wilted (about 2 minutes). Reduce heat to very low, to keep warm. Combine olive oil, salt and pepper, mashed garlic, and capers. Rub mixture into both sides of salmon steaks. Grill the fish or broil 3–4 inches from flame for 2–2 ½ minutes on each side. Set fish aside. Remove spinach from heat and toss with vinegar; divide equally on 4 plates. Add grilled salmon fillet to bed of spinach on each plate and garnish with onions. Serve.

Approx. 250 calories per serving
18g protein, 8g total fat, 1g saturated fat, 0 trans fat,
14g carbohydrates, 188mg cholesterol, 884mg sodium, 6g fiber

Chicken Piccata
(MAKES 4 SERVINGS)

2 teaspoons extra-virgin olive oil
4 (3-ounce) skinless, boneless chicken breast fillets, lightly pounded
Salt and freshly ground pepper to taste
3 cloves fresh garlic, minced
1 cup low-sodium, fat-free chicken broth
2 tablespoons dry white wine
4 teaspoons lemon juice
1 tablespoon all-purpose flour
2 tablespoons chopped fresh parsley
1 tablespoon capers
Lemon wedges for garnish

Rinse chicken breast fillets under cold water and pat dry, then place breasts between layers of wax paper and lightly pound fillets with a meat mallet. Lightly sprinkle each fillet with salt and pepper if desired. Heat 1 teaspoon of olive oil in a large heavy-bottomed skillet over medium heat, add chicken fillets, and cook until fillets are lightly browned and centers cooked (juice will run clear). Transfer fillets to a serving platter and put in a low-temperature oven to keep warm. Add remaining teaspoon of oil and garlic to skillet and cook for 30 seconds to soften. Combine chicken broth, wine, lemon juice, and flour in skillet where chicken was cooked. Stir to blend, and continue stirring until mixture thickens. Add parsley and capers to sauce. Remove chicken from oven, place each fillet on a plate, and spoon mixture over fillets. Garnish with lemon wedges. Serve with cooked spinach linguine or pasta of choice.

Approx. 223 calories per serving
21g protein, 11g total fat, 2g saturated fat, 0 trans fat,
4g carbohydrates, 48mg cholesterol, 380mg sodium, <0.5g fiber

Spicy Whole Wheat Capellini with Garlic
(MAKES 4 SERVINGS)

8 ounces whole wheat capellini pasta
¼ cup extra-virgin olive oil
4 cloves garlic, chopped
1 teaspoon diced hot peppers
Salt and fresh ground pepper to taste
Grated Pecorino or Parmesan cheese (optional)

Bring water to a boil, add pasta, and cook pasta until al dente. Remove from heat, drain pasta, and return to pot, drizzling with scant amount of olive oil to keep pasta from sticking together. Set aside. In a heavy skillet over medium heat, add olive oil, then sauté garlic and hot pepper until tender (about 1–2 minutes). Add to pasta and toss. Add salt and pepper to taste, and sprinkle with grated cheese if desired.

Approx. 299 calories per serving
8g protein, 16g total fat, 2g saturated fat, 0 trans fat,
35g carbohydrates, 4mg cholesterol, 0 sodium, 7g fiber

Fettuccine with Smoked Salmon and Basil Pesto
(MAKES 4 SERVINGS)

8 ounces dried whole grain fettuccine pasta
Drizzle of extra-virgin olive oil
¼ cup Market fresh pesto
10 pitted black olives, halved
½ tablespoon capers, rinsed well and drained
6 ounces nova smoked salmon (cut into thin strips)
1 tablespoon freshly grated Romano cheese
4 sprigs fresh basil leaves for garnish

Bring water to a boil, add pasta, and cook pasta until al dente. Remove
from heat, drain pasta, and return to pot, drizzling with scant amount
of olive oil to keep pasta from sticking together. Set aside. Meanwhile,
warm pesto sauce in a saucepan under low heat, add olives and capers,
remove from heat and add salmon. In a large serving bowl, toss pasta
with salmon mixture. Divide into 4 portions, and serve with ¼ tablespoon of cheese, garnished with a fresh basil sprig.

Approx. 323 calories per serving
15g protein, 10g total fat, 2g saturated fat, 0 trans fat,
44g carbohydrates, 14mg cholesterol, 540mg sodium, <1g fiber

Baked Tilapia
(MAKES 2 SERVINGS)

4 (4-ounce) tilapia fillets
2 tablespoons extra-virgin olive oil
3 cloves garlic, minced
2 scallions, white and green parts, chopped
½ cup fresh chopped parsley
Salt and freshly ground pepper to taste
Fresh spinach leaves and 6 grape tomatoes, halved, for garnish

Juice from 2 lemons
1 lemon, quartered

Rinse fillets under cold water and pat dry. Place fillets in a baking dish. In mixing bowl combine oil, garlic, scallions, and parsley; pour over fish, cover, and refrigerate for 30 minutes. Sprinkle with salt and pepper and bake at 350 degrees for 15 minutes or until fish flakes easily. Divide cleaned spinach on 2 plates. Remove fish from oven, and place 2 fillets on top of spinach on each plate. Garnish each plate with tomato halves. Squeeze juice from 2 lemons over fillets, garnish with lemon wedge, and serve.

Approx. 138 calories per serving (two fillets per serving)
15g protein, 8g total fat, 1g saturated fat, 0 trans fat,
3g carbohydrates, 43mg cholesterol, 46mg sodium, 0 fiber

Fettuccine with Sundried Tomatoes and Goat Cheese
(MAKES 6–8 SERVINGS)

4 tablespoons chopped sundried tomatoes (in olive oil)
1 cup sliced scallions
4 garlic cloves, minced
1 medium red bell pepper, thinly sliced
½ cup dry vermouth
¼ cup chopped fresh basil
10 pitted Kalamata olives
1 tablespoon capers, rinsed and drained
2 teaspoons dried oregano
1 pound whole wheat fettuccine, cooked and drained
6 ounces low-fat goat cheese, crumbled

Drain oil from tomatoes and reserve oil; set tomatoes aside. In a large skillet, heat oil from tomatoes over medium heat. Add scallions and garlic to oil and sauté until soft. Add red peppers and ¼ cup of vermouth to garlic mixture. Cook peppers until crispy tender or until vermouth is almost evaporated. Reduce heat to simmer, and add tomatoes, remaining ¼ cup of vermouth, basil, olives, capers, and oregano. Simmer, stirring often to incorporate flavors (about 5–8 minutes), then reduce to very low heat to keep warm. Cook pasta to desired consistency (al dente would be best), and drain. Place pasta in a large bowl and toss with goat cheese until well blended. Add tomato mixture and toss again until well mixed. Serve.

Approx. 269 calories per serving
12g protein, 6g total fat, 2g saturated fat, 0 trans fat,
44g carbohydrates, 4mg cholesterol, 323mg sodium, 7g fiber

SIDE DISHES

Grilled Eggplant
(MAKES 4 SERVINGS)

1 tablespoon extra-virgin olive oil
2 tablespoons fresh oregano leaves
2 plum tomatoes, diced
1½ pounds eggplant, cut lengthwise into ½-inch thick slices
Olive oil cooking spray
2 large garlic cloves, finely minced
1 teaspoon chopped dried rosemary
¼ teaspoon freshly ground pepper
¼ cup crumbled feta cheese
Lemon wedges
Oregano sprigs for garnish
Salt and freshly ground pepper to taste

Heat oil in saucepan, add oregano leaves, then remove pan from heat. Add tomato to oregano and allow to bathe in hot oil until ready to serve. Meanwhile, spray both sides of eggplant with olive oil spray, sprinkle with garlic, rosemary, and salt and pepper, and place on medium-hot grill. Cover grill and cook eggplant until tender and browned on both sides, turning once. Remove eggplant to platter, drizzle with oregano tomato oil, and top with feta cheese. Garnish with lemon wedges and oregano sprigs.

Approx. 74 calories per serving
4g protein, 6g total fat, 1g saturated fat, 0 trans fat,
10g carbohydrates, 5mg cholesterol, 86mg sodium, 0.2g fiber

Roasted Peppers
(MAKES 4–6 SERVINGS)

4 large red bell peppers
2 cloves garlic, peeled and sliced
4 tablespoons extra-virgin olive oil
Salt and freshly ground pepper to taste

Clean peppers and pat dry. Place peppers on moderately hot grill or on a rack under a broiler 1–2 inches from heat, turning often until skin is charred and blistered. Charring of entire skin takes about 15–20 minutes. Remove from grill or broiler and place peppers aside to cool. When cool enough to handle, rub off blackened skins. Cut each pepper in half, remove stalk and seeds, and cut into ½-inch strips. Place strips in a bowl, and add garlic, oil, and salt and pepper to taste. Toss and set aside for about 30 minutes before serving.

Approx. 108 calories per serving
1g protein, 10g total fat, 1g saturated fat, 0 trans fat,
7g carbohydrates, 0 cholesterol, 2mg sodium, 2g fiber

Broccoli with Fresh Garlic
(MAKES 4–6 SERVINGS)

10–12 fresh broccoli spears, roughly 6 inches long
3 cups low-sodium, fat-free chicken broth
3 tablespoons extra-virgin olive oil
2–3 cloves fresh garlic, crushed
2 tablespoons chopped fresh parsley
Salt to taste
Pinch of freshly ground pepper

Cook spears in a large skillet of low-salt chicken broth until slightly undercooked (about 7 minutes). Test with a fork; do not overcook. Drain well and set aside. Heat oil in a large skillet over medium-high heat; add garlic and sauté until golden brown. Add broccoli, parsley, and seasoning to taste. Turn broccoli several times, mixing well with seasonings, oil, and garlic. Serve immediately.

Approx. 161 calories per serving
11g protein, 9g total fat, 2g saturated fat, 0 trans fat,
16g carbohydrates, 1mg cholesterol, 80mg sodium, 9g fiber

DESSERTS

Drunken Apricots
(MAKES 4 SERVINGS)

8 medium apricots
1½ cups red wine
1 ⅓ cups water
3 strips lemon peel (yellow part only)
3 tablespoons honey
1 cinnamon stick
Sprinkle with non-caloric sweetener to taste (optional)
Fat-free whipped cream (optional)

Peel skin from apricots. In a saucepan add wine, water, lemon peel, honey, and cinnamon stick, and bring to boil. Add apricots to sauce, submerging under liquid as much as possible, and gently poach for 5–10 minutes, until just tender. Remove apricots from saucepan and place in a bowl; set aside. Boil liquid in the saucepan, stirring constantly, until it becomes thick and syrupy. Remove cinnamon stick and lemon peel before liquid becomes dark. Pour syrup, when cool, over apricots, and serve. Garnish with sweetener and whipped cream if desired.

Approx. 112 calories per serving
1g protein, 0.3g total fat, 0 saturated fat, 0 trans fat,
20g carbohydrates, 0 cholesterol, 1mg sodium, 1g fiber

Strawberries and Balsamic Syrup
(MAKES 4 SERVINGS)

2 ½ cups strawberries, hulled and halved
4 tablespoons Crème de Banana liqueur
non-caloric sweetener to taste
Balsamic syrup

Combine strawberries and liqueur in a large bowl, toss well, cover, and refrigerate 20–30 minutes. When ready to serve, remove strawberries with a slotted spoon and place in a single layer on a dessert platter. Dust generously with sweetener, drizzle with balsamic syrup, and serve.

Approx. 49 calories per serving
<1g protein, 0.4g total fat, <0.1g saturated fat, 0 trans fat,
7g carbohydrates, 0 cholesterol, 1mg sodium, 2g fiber

Honeydew Sorbet
(MAKES 4–6 SERVINGS)

1½ cups of water
½ cup low-calorie baking sweetener
2 ripe honeydews (about 5 inches in diameter each), peeled, seeded, and chunked
¼ cup fresh lemon juice
¼ cup egg whites
Mint sprigs for garnish

Combine water and sweetener, and bring to a boil over medium heat. Reduce heat and simmer for 5 minutes, then allow to cool. In a food processor or blender add honeydew and its juices, lemon juice, and cooled syrup. Puree until smooth. Pour mixture into bowl and freeze until almost frozen. Remove from freezer and beat with an electric beater until mixture is again smooth. Beat egg white until stiff and fold into frozen fruit mixture. Cover container and freeze again until firm (about 2–3 hours). When ready to serve, scoop into dessert cups and garnish with mint sprig if desired.

Approx. 117 calories per serving
2g protein, <0.5g total fat, 0 saturated fat, 0 trans fat,
31g carbohydrates, 0 cholesterol, 33mg sodium, 2g fiber

Meringue Cookies
(MAKES 20–24 COOKIES)

1 cup liquid egg whites
Pinch of cream of tartar
¼ cup low-calorie baking sweetener
1 teaspoon white wine vinegar
1 teaspoon vanilla extract

Line 2 cookie trays with parchment paper. Place egg whites in a mixing bowl and slowly whisk on low speed with an electric beater until they begin to bubble. Add cream of tartar and increase speed slightly; whisk until the mixture begins to peak. Increase speed to medium and slowly add sweetener, vinegar, and vanilla extract. Continue whisking until mixture is satiny and firmly holds peak. Ladle a soup spoon-sized portion of mixture onto parchment-lined trays to make 20–24 cookies. Put trays of meringues in an oven preheated to 275 degrees to bake for about 1 hour. Turn off oven and allow cookies to stand in closed oven for an additional hour to dry. When meringues are pierced with a toothpick that comes back dry, they are ready. Transfer cookies to cooling racks to continue to cool.

Approx. 5 calories per cookie
1g protein, 0 total fat, 0 saturated fat, 0 trans fat,
<0.1g carbohydrates, 0 cholesterol, 15mg sodium, 0 fiber

Sweet Plum Compote
(MAKES 6 SERVINGS)

Canola oil cooking spray
3 lbs. ripe plums, halved and pitted
¼ cup low-calorie baking sweetener
1 cup water
1 tablespoon Crème de Cassis liqueur

Lightly spray a baking dish with cooking spray. Add plums to baking dish. Combine sweetener and water in a saucepan and bring to a boil; cook for about 5 minutes, stirring constantly, or until liquid becomes syrupy. Pour syrup over plums and drizzle with Crème de Cassis. Bake mixture for 45 minutes to 1 hour in a 350-degree oven. Serve warm or cool.

Approx. 130 calories per serving
2g protein, 1g total fat, 0.1g saturated fat, 0 trans fat
28g carbohydrates, 0 cholesterol, 1mg sodium, 1g fiber

Peach Marsala Compote
(MAKES 6 SERVINGS)

Canola oil cooking spray
12 fresh peaches
6 cups water
¾ cup low-calorie baking sweetener
½ cup Marsala wine
½ teaspoon ground cinnamon
½ teaspoon vanilla extract
½ teaspoon freshly grated nutmeg

Lightly spray a 2-quart baking dish with cooking spray. Blanch the peaches in boiling water for 20 seconds, then remove skin while holding under cold running water. Pit and slice peaches. Add peaches, sweetener, wine, cinnamon, vanilla extract, and nutmeg to a baking dish and bake for 45 minutes to 1 hour in a 350-degree oven. Serve warm or at room temperature.

Approx. 80 calories per serving
1g protein, 0.2g total fat, 0 saturated fat, 0 trans fat,
21g carbohydrates, 0 cholesterol, 126mg sodium, 3g fiber

Strawberries Amaretto
(MAKES 8 SERVINGS)

3 pints of fresh strawberries
2 cups plain low-fat yogurt
1 teaspoon vanilla extract
¼ cup Amaretto liqueur
Fat-free whipped cream (if desired)

Set aside 8 strawberries for garnish. Hull remaining strawberries and cut into halves. Place strawberry halves in dessert cups. In a bowl combine yogurt, vanilla extract, and liqueur; blend well. Pour over strawberries and garnish each cup with a reserved berry. Add whipped cream if desired.

Approx. 96 calories per serving

4g protein, 0.6g total fat, <0.5 saturated fat, 0 trans fat,

9g carbohydrates, <0.5mg cholesterol, 42mg sodium, 3g fiber

Fresh Fruit Kebobs and Cinnamon Honey Dip
(MAKES 2 SERVINGS)

Assorted bite-sized chunks of your favorite fresh fruits (enough for 2
*   8-inch wooden skewers)*
1 cup of low-fat plain yogurt
2 tablespoons of honey or non-caloric sweetener
Pinch of ground white pepper
6 teaspoons of ground cinnamon or to taste

Prepare fruits on skewers and set aside. Combine yogurt, honey, and white pepper, and mix well. Divide mixture into two individual serving bowls; sprinkle cinnamon on top of each serving and gently swirl in. Cover and refrigerate to chill before serving. NOTE: Values shown are for yogurt dip only (values for fruit cannot be calculated since they depend on the specific fruits chosen).

Approx. 70 calories per serving

0.5g protein, 2g total fat, 1g saturated fat, 0 trans fat,

8g carbohydrates, 7mg cholesterol, 75mg sodium, 0 fiber

The Restaurant Survival Guide

THERE'S NO QUESTION that cooking your food at home is the best way to ensure that what you are eating is heart-healthy. But does that mean you never get to go out to a restaurant? Not at all!

You can take heart-healthy nutrition on the road and have a wonderful—and healthy—time. Just use these easy-to-follow recommendations:

1. Never go to a restaurant when you are starving. Drink a glass of water and enjoy a handful of almonds before you go. That way you won't be tempted to devour everything in the bread basket while you're waiting for your meal.

2. Speaking of that bread basket, ask for whole grain bread and olive oil if white bread and butter arrives. But if you're watching your calories, remember, a tablespoon of olive oil has 120 calories, so drizzle, don't pour. You can also mix it with a little balsamic vinegar if desired.

3. Order a salad to start, and for a dressing, request olive oil and vinegar on the side. Believe me, you won't miss that heavy ranch or processed Thousand Island.

4. For your main dish, choose fish or skinless poultry over red meat, and don't forget a side of vegetables.

5. Choose foods that are baked, broiled, or grilled—never fried.

6. Steer clear of processed foods. Fresh food is always healthier, and it tastes much better too!

7. Be certain your foods are not being cooked with trans fats (partially hydrogenated oils). Don't be afraid to ask your server!

8. When ordering pasta, ask for a whole grain version. Most restaurants will have one.

9. Choose brown rice over white rice.

10. Avoid fruit drinks and sodas. Unsweetened iced tea, especially green tea, is always a good option if you want a change from water.

11. Eat half of your portion and take the rest home. You can even ask for half of your portion to be wrapped up ahead of time!

12. Order fresh fruit for dessert.

13. Complete your meal with a hot green tea.

Appendix E

National Cholesterol Guidelines

ATP III At-A-Glance

Detection, Evaluation, and Treatment of High Blood Cholesterol in Adults
(Reprinted with Permission of the National Cholesterol Education Program)

TABLE OF CONTENTS

STEP 1: Determine lipoprotein levels—obtain complete lipoprotein profile after 9- to 12-hour fast

STEP 2: Identify presence of clinical atherosclerotic disease that confers high risk for coronary heart disease (CHD) events (CHD risk equivalent)

STEP 3: Determine presence of major risk factors (other than LDL)

STEP 4: If 2+ risk factors (other than LDL) are present without CHD or CHD risk equivalent, assess 10-year (short-term) CHD risk

STEP 5: Determine risk category

STEP 6: Initiate therapeutic lifestyle changes (TLC) if LDL is above goal

STEP 7: Consider adding drug therapy if LDL exceeds levels shown in Step 5 table

STEP 8: Identify metabolic syndrome and treat, if present, after 3 months of TLC

STEP 9: Treat elevated triglycerides

STEP 1: Determine lipoprotein levels—obtain complete lipoprotein profile after 9- to 12-hour fast.

ATP III Classification of LDL, Total, and HDL Cholesterol (mg/dL)

LDL Cholesterol - Primary Target of Therapy

<100	Optimal
100–129	Near Optimal/Above Optimal
130–159	Borderline High
160–189	High
≥190	Very high

Total Cholesterol

<200	Desirable
200–239	Borderline High
≥240	High

HDL Cholesterol

<40	Low
≥60	High

STEP 2: Identify presence of clinical atherosclerotic disease that confers high risk for coronary heart disease (CHD) events (CHD risk equivalent).

- Clinical CHD
- Symptomatic carotid artery disease
- Peripheral arterial disease
- Abdominal aortic aneurysm

STEP 3: Determine presence of major risk factors (other than LDL).

Major Risk Factors (Exclusive of LDL Cholesterol) That Modify LDL Goals
- Cigarette smoking
- Hypertension (BP ≥140/90 mmHg or on antihypertensive medication)
- Low HDL cholesterol (<40 mg/dl)*
- Family history of premature CHD (CHD in male first degree relative <55 years; CHD in female first degree relative <65 years)
- Age (men ≥45 years; women ≥55 years)

* HDL cholesterol ≥60 mg/dL counts as a "negative" risk factor; its presence removes one risk factor from the total count.

NOTE: In ATP III, diabetes is regarded as a CHD risk equivalent.

STEP 4: If 2+ risk factors (other than LDL) are present without CHD or CHD risk equivalent, assess 10-year (short-term) CHD risk (see Framingham tables).

Three levels of 10-year risk:
- >20% (CHD risk equivalent)
- 10–20%
- <10%

STEP 5: Determine risk category.

Establish LDL goal of therapy
- Determine need for therapeutic lifestyle changes (TLC)
- Determine level for drug consideration
- LDL cholesterol goals and cutpoints for therapeutic lifestyle changes (TLC) and drug therapy in different risk categories

Risk Category	LDL Goal	LDL Level at Which to Initiate Therapeutic Lifestyle Changes (TLC)	LDL Level at Which to Consider Drug Therapy
CHD or CHD Risk Equivalents (10-year risk >20%)	<100 mg/dL	≥100 mg/dL	≥130 mg/dL (100–129 mg/dL: drug optional)*
2+ Risk Factors (10-year risk ≤20%)	<130 mg/dL	≥130 mg/dL	10-year risk 10–20%: ≥130 mg/dL 10-year risk <10%: ≥160 mg/dL
0–1 Risk Factor**	<160 mg/dL	≥160 mg/dL	≥190 mg/dL (160–189 mg/dL: LDL-lowering drug optional)

* Some authorities recommend use of LDL-lowering drugs in this category if an LDL cholesterol <100 mg/dL cannot be achieved by therapeutic lifestyle changes. Others prefer use of drugs that primarily modify triglycerides and HDL, e.g., nicotinic acid or fibrate. Clinical judgment also may call for deferring drug therapy in this subcategory.
** Almost all people with 0–1 risk factor have a 10-year risk <10%, thus 10-year risk assessment in people with 0–1 risk factor is not necessary.

STEP 6: Initiate therapeutic lifestyle changes (TLC) if LDL is above goal.

TLC Features
- TLC Diet:
- Saturated fat <7% of calories, cholesterol <200 mg/day
- Consider increased viscous (soluble) fiber (10–25 g/ day) and plant stanols/sterols (2g/day) as therapeutic options to enhance LDL lowering
- Weight management
- Increased physical activity

STEP 7: Consider adding drug therapy if LDL exceeds levels shown in Step 5 table.

- Consider drug simultaneously with TLC for CHD and CHD equivalents.
- Consider adding drug to TLC after 3 months for other risk categories.

Drugs Affecting Lipoprotein Metabolism

Drug Class	Agents and Daily Doses	Lipid/ Lipoprotein Effects	Side Effects	Contraindications
HMG CoA reductase inhibitors (statins)	Lovastatin (20-80 mg), Pravastatin (20–40 mg), Simvastatin (20–80 mg), Fluvastatin (20–80 mg), Atorvastatin (10–80 mg), Cerivastatin (0.4–0.8 mg)	LDL-C 18–55% HDL-C 5–15% TG 7–30%	Myopathy Increased liver enzymes	Absolute: • Active or chronic liver disease Relative: • Concomitant use of certain drugs*
Bile acid equestrants	Cholestyramine (4–16 g) Colestipol (5–20 g) Colesevelam (2.6–3.8 g)	LDL-C 15–30% HDL-C 3–5% TG No change or increase	Gastrointestinal distress Constipation Decreased absorption of other drugs	Absolute: • dysbetalipo- proteinemia • TG >400 mg/ dL Relative: • TG >200 mg/ dL
Nicotinic acid	Immediate release (crystalline) nicotinic acid (1.5–3 gm), extended release nicotinic acid (Niaspan ®) (1–2 g), sustained release nicotinic acid (1–2 g)	LDL-C 5–25% HDL-C 15–35% TG 20–50%	Flushing Hyperglycemia Hyperuricemia (or gout) Upper GI distress Hepatotoxicity	Absolute: • Chronic liver disease • Severe gout Relative: • Diabetes • Hyperuricemia • Peptic ulcer disease
Fibric acids	Gemfibrozil (600 mg BID) Fenofibrate (200 mg) Clofibrate (1000 mg BID)	LDL-C 5–20% (may be increased in patients with high TG) HDL-C 10–20% TG 20–50%	Dyspepsia Gallstones Myopathy	Absolute: • Severe renal disease • Severe hepatic disease

* Cyclosporine, macrolide antibiotics, various anti-fungal agents, and cytochrome P-450 inhibitors (fibrates and niacin should be used with appropriate caution).

STEP 8: Identify metabolic syndrome and treat, if present, after 3 months of TLC.

Clinical Identification of Metabolic Syndrome—Any 3 of the Following:

Risk Factor	Defining Level
Abdominal obesity* Men Women	Waist circumference** >102 cm (>40 in) >88 cm (>35 in)
Triglycerides	≥150 mg/dL
HDL cholesterol Men Women	 <40 mg/dl <50 mg/dl
blood pressure	≥130/≥85 mmHg
Fasting glucose	≥110 mg/dL

* Overweight and obesity are associated with insulin resistance and metabolic syndrome. However, the presence of abdominal obesity is more highly correlated with metabolic risk factors than is an elevated body mass index (BMI). Therefore, the simple measure of waist circumference is recommended to identify the body weight component of metabolic syndrome.

** Some male patients can develop multiple metabolic risk factors when the waist circumference is only marginally increased, e.g., 94–102 cm (37–39 in). Such patients may have a strong genetic contribution to insulin resistance. They should benefit from changes in life habits, similarly to men with categorical increases in waist circumference.

Treatment of Metabolic Syndrome

- Treat underlying causes (overweight/obesity and physical inactivity):
- Intensify weight management
- Increase physical activity
- Treat lipid and non-lipid risk factors if they persist despite these lifestyle therapies:
- Treat hypertension
- Use aspirin for CHD patients to reduce prothrombotic state
- Treat elevated triglycerides and/or low HDL (as shown in Step 9 below)

STEP 9: Treat elevated triglycerides.

ATP III Classification of Serum Triglycerides (mg/dL)

< 150	Normal
150–199	Borderline high
200–499	High
≥500	Very high

Treatment of Elevated Triglycerides (≥150 mg/dL)
- Primary aim of therapy is to reach LDL goal
- Intensify weight management
- Increase physical activity
- If triglycerides are ≥200 mg/dL after LDL goal is reached, set secondary goal for non-HDL cholesterol (total - HDL) 30 mg/dL higher than LDL goal

Comparison of LDL Cholesterol and Non-HDL Cholesterol Goals for Three Risk Categories=

Risk Category	LDL Goal (mg/dL)	Non-HDL Goal (mg/dL)
CHD and CHD Risk Equivalent (10-year risk for CHD >20%)	<100	<130
Multiple (2+) Risk Factors and 10-year risk ≤20%	<130	<160
0-1 Risk Factor	<160	<190

If triglycerides 200–499 mg/dL after LDL goal is reached, consider adding drug if needed to reach non-HDL goal:
- Intensify therapy with LDL-lowering drug, or
- Add nicotinic acid or fibrate to further lower VLDL

If triglycerides ≥500 mg/dL, first lower triglycerides to prevent pancreatitis:
- Very low-fat diet (≤15% of calories from fat)
- Weight management and physical activity
- Fibrate or nicotinic acid
- When triglycerides <500 mg/dL, turn to LDL-lowering therapy

Treatment of low HDL cholesterol (<40 mg/dL)
- First reach LDL goal, then:
- Intensify weight management and increase physical activity
- If triglycerides 200–499 mg/dL, achieve non-HDL goal
- If triglycerides <200 mg/dL (isolated low HDL) in CHD or CHD equivalent, consider nicotinic acid or fibrate

U.S. DEPARTMENT OF HEALTH AND HUMAN SERVICES
Public Health Service—National Institutes of Health
National Heart, Lung, and Blood Institute. NIH Publication No. 01-3305. May 2001

Advanced Cardiovascular Diagnostic Tests

Much of the progress in the diagnosis and treatment of cardiovascular disease can be attributed to the discovery of new biomarkers. These biomarkers, which can be measured with a blood test, give healthcare providers a greater insight into heart disease risk than simply looking at a standard cholesterol panel. Indeed, advanced diagnostic laboratory tests help to uncover "hidden risks" for heart attack so that proper treatment with lifestyle intervention and medical therapy can be initiated.

The following sample lab report and explanation of the blood test results has been provided courtesy of Health Diagnostic Laboratory.

(For even more, regularly updated information regarding biomarkers and heart attack prevention, visit www.drozner.com.)

HealthDiagnosticLaboratoryInc.
beyond disease diagnosis

Laboratory Results

Patient

| Name: | Phone #: | Patient ID #: |
| Test M Smith | (678) 555-1212 | 12346 |

| Fasting Status: | Gender: | Birthdate: | Age: |
| 12 hours | Male | 8/12/1928 | 83 |

| Height: | Weight: | BMI: | Prev. BMI: 9/29/201 |
| 5 ft 11 in | 200 lbs | 28 | 28 |

Specimen

| Collection Time: | Specimen ID: |
| 2:38 pm | 10022300198 |

| Collection Date: | Report Type: |
| 5/6/2011 | Complete |

| Received Date: | Report Date: |
| 5/6/2002 | 9/29/2011 |

Provider

Requesting Provider:
Bob Johnson, MD
ABC Family Practice
123 Broad St., Suite 456
Richmond, VA 12345

Client ID:
11-22222-33-4444444

Laboratory Test	Notes	High Risk	Intermediate Risk	Optimal	High Risk Range	Intermediate Risk Range	Optimal Range	Previous Results 9/29/2011
Lipids								
Total Cholesterol (mg/dL)				200	≥ 240	200 - 239	< 200	29
LDL-C Direct (mg/dL)		135			≥ 130 CHD & CHD risk eq. > 100	100 - 129 CHD & CHD risk eq. 70 - 100	< 100 CHD & CHD risk eq. < 70	23
HDL-C (mg/dL)				70	< 40		≥ 40	51
Triglycerides (mg/dL)				100	≥ 200	150 - 199	< 150	
Non-HDL-C (mg/dL) (calculated)				110	≥ 160	130 - 159	< 130	
Lipoprotein Particles and Apolipoproteins								
Apo B (mg/dL)		85			≥ 80	60 - 79	< 60	55
LDL-P (nmol/L)				1100	≥ 1300	1000 - 1299	< 1000	1850
sdLDL (mg/dL)*				30	≥ 31	21 - 30	≤ 20	
% sdLDL (calculated)				15	> 30	26 - 30	< 26	
Apo A-I (mg/dL)		113			< 114	114 - 131	≥ 132	
HDL-P (µmol/L)		25.0			< 28.0	28.0 - 34.0	≥ 35.0	
HDL2 (mg/dL)*				10	≤ 8	9 - 11	≥ 12	2
Apo B:Apo A-I Ratio (calculated)				0.42	≥ 0.81	0.61 - 0.81	≤ 0.6	
Lp(a) Mass (mg/dL)				< 12	≥ 30		< 30	42
Lp(a) Cholesterol (mg/dL)		8			≥ 6	3 - 5	< 3	30
Inflammation/Oxidation								
Myeloperoxidase (pmol/L)				120	≥ 550	400 - 549	< 400	
Lp-PLA₂ (ng/mL)		240			> 235	200 - 235	< 200	
hs-CRP (mg/L)		3.2			≥ 3.0	1.0 - 2.9	< 1.0	
Fibrinogen (mg/dL)				300	≥ 465	391 - 464	≤ 390	
F₂-Isoprostanes (urine) (ng/mg of creatinine)				0.80	> 1.00		0.10 - 1.00	
Myocardial Stress								
NT-proBNP (pg/mL)				400	≥ 450	125 - 449	< 125	
Galectin-3 (ng/mL)				8.0	> 25.9	17.9 - 25.9	≤ 17.8	

Lab Notes: Result revised from: 2.3. Result revised from: 1.3. Result revised from: 0.3. QNS. Lorem ipsum dolor sit amet, consectetur adipisicing elit, sed do eiusmod tempor incididunt ut labore et dolore magna aliqua. Ut enim ad minim veniam, quis nostrud exercitation ullamco laboris nisi ut aliquip ex ea commodo consequat. Duis aute irure dolor in reprehenderit in voluptate velit

Provider Notes:

www.myhdl.com

or visit us online at www.myhdl.com (1-877-443-5227) or call 1-877-4HDLABS please call 1-877-4HDLABS (1-877-443-5227) To schedule time with a Personal Health Coach,

Dr. Joseph P. McConnell | Laboratory Director | CLIA No. 49D1100708 | CAP No. 7224971 | NPI No. 1629209853
©2010 | 737 N. 5th Street Suite 103 | Richmond, Virginia 23219 | Phone: 804.343.2718 | Fax: 804.343.2704

HDL 20.0

HealthDiagnosticLaboratoryInc.
beyond disease diagnosis

Laboratory Results

Patient

Name:	Phone #:	Patient ID #:
Test M Smith	(678) 555-1212	12346

Fasting Status:	Gender:	Birthdate:	Age:
12 hours	Male	8/12/1928	83

Height:	Weight:	BMI:		Prev. BMI: 9/29/201	
5 ft 11 in	200 lbs		28		28

Specimen

Collection Time:	Specimen ID:
2:38 pm	10022300198

Collection Date:	Report Type:
5/6/2011	Complete

Received Date:	Report Date:
5/6/2002	9/29/2011

Provider

Requesting Provider:
Bob Johnson, MD
ABC Family Practice
123 Broad St., Suite 456
Richmond, VA 12345

Client ID:
11-22222-33-4444444

Laboratory Test	Notes	High Risk	Intermediate Risk	Optimal	High Risk Range	Intermediate Risk Range	Optimal Range	Previous Results 9/29/2011
Platelets AspirinWorks® (urine) (pg/mg of creatinine)				500	> 1500		≤ 1500	
Lipoprotein Genetics Apolipoprotein E Genotype*		3/4			Estimated Genotype Frequency: 2/2 (~1-2%), 2/3 (~15%), 2/4 (~1-2%), 3/3 (~55%), 3/4 (~25%), 4/4 (~1-2%)			
Platelet Genetics CYP2C19*2*3* Poor metabolizers with poor antiplatelet effect of Plavix.		*2/*3			*1/*1 = optimal, *1/*2 or *1/*3 = intermediate, *2/*2, *2/*3 or *3/*3 = poor			*2/*2
CYP2C19*17* Rapid metabolizers at increased risk for bleeding on Plavix.			*1/*17		*1/*1 = optimal, *1/*17 = rapid, *17/*17 = ultra rapid			Not Tested
Coagulation Genetics Factor V Leiden		Arg/Gln			Optimal=Non-carrier (Arg/Arg); At Risk=(Arg/Gln or Gln/Gln)			
Prothrombin Mutation				G/G	Optimal=Non-carrier (G/G); At Risk=(G/A or A/A)			
MTHFR (Methylenetetrahydrofolate Reductase)		T/T			Estimated Genotype Frequency: C/C (~49.3%), C/T (~39.8%), T/T (~10.9%)			C/C
CYP2C9*2*				C/C	Warfarin metabolism: C/C = normal, C/T = intermediate, T/T = poor			
CYP2C9*3*			C/A		Warfarin metabolism: A/A = normal, C/A = intermediate, C/C = poor			
VKORC1 3673		A/A			Warfarin response: G/G = poor, G/A = intermediate, A/A = extensive			

Lab Notes: Result revised from: 2.3. Result revised from: 1.3. Result revised from: 0.3. QNS. Lorem ipsum dolor sit amet, consectetur adipisicing elit, sed do eiusmod tempor incididunt ut labore et dolore magna aliqua. Ut enim ad minim veniam, quis nostrud exercitation ullamco laboris nisi ut aliquip ex ea commodo consequat. Duis aute irure dolor in reprehenderit in voluptate velit esse cillum dolore eu fugiat nulla pariatur. Excepteur sint occaecat cupidatat non proident, sunt in culpa qui officia deserunt mollit anim id est laborum.

Dr. Joseph P. McConnell | Laboratory Director | CLIA No. 49D1100708 | CAP No. 7224971 | NPI No. 1629209853
©2010 | 737 N. 5th Street Suite 103 | Richmond, Virginia 23219 | Phone: 804.343.2718 | Fax: 804.343.2704

HDL 20.0

To schedule time with a Personal Health Coach, please call 1-877-4HDLABS (1-877-443-5227) or visit us online at www.myhdi.com

HealthDiagnosticLaboratoryInc.
beyond disease diagnosis

Laboratory Results

Patient

Name:	Test M Smith
Phone #:	(678) 555-1212
Patient ID #:	12346
Fasting Status:	12 hours
Gender:	Male
Birthdate:	8/12/1928
Age:	83
Height:	5 ft 11 in
Weight:	200 lbs
BMI:	28
Prev. BMI 9/29/201:	28

Specimen

Collection Time:	2:38 pm
Specimen ID:	10022300198
Collection Date:	5/6/2011
Report Type:	Complete
Received Date:	5/6/2002
Report Date:	9/29/2011

Provider

Requesting Provider:
Bob Johnson, MD
ABC Family Practice
123 Broad St., Suite 456
Richmond, VA 12345
Client ID:
11-22222-33-4444444

Laboratory Test	Notes	High Risk	Intermediate Risk	Optimal	High Risk Range	Intermediate Risk Range	Optimal Range	Previous Results 9/29/2011
Metabolic								
Insulin (µU/mL)		14			≥ 12	10 - 11	3 - 9	
C-peptide (ng/mL)				1.2	≤ 1.0 or > 4.4		1.1 - 4.4	
Free Fatty Acid (mmol/L)				0.10	> 0.7	0.6 - 0.7	≤ 0.59	
Glucose (mg/dL)				74	≤ 55 or > 125	56-69 or 100-125	70 - 99	
HbA1c (%)				3.6	≥ 6.5	5.7 - 6.4	≤ 5.6	
Estimated Average Glucose (mg/dL) (calculated)		142.3			≥ 139.9	116.9 - 139.8	≤ 116.8	
25-hydroxy-Vitamin D (ng/mL)		12			≤ 14	15 - 29	30 - 100	
Uric Acid (mg/dL)				6.2	≥ 8	7.0 - 7.9	3.4 - 6.9	
TSH (µIU/mL)		4.30			< 0.27 or > 4.20		0.27 - 4.20	
Homocysteine (µmol/L)			12		> 13	11 - 13	≤ 10	
Vitamin B₁₂ (pg/mL)			256		< 211	211 - 299	≥ 300	
RBC Folate (ng/mL)		264			≤ 467		≥ 468	
Renal								
Cystatin C (mg/L)		1.11			≥ 1.04	0.96 - 1.03	≤ 0.95	
Estimated Glomerular Filtration Rate (eGFR, mL/min/1.73m2)		61			≤ 79	80 - 124	≥ 125	
Microalbumin (urine) (mg albumin/g of creatinine)				12	≥ 20		≤ 19	
Creatinine, serum (mg/dL)				0.8	> 1.2		0.7 - 1.2	

Lab Notes: Result revised from: 2.3. Result revised from: 1.3. Result revised from: 0.3. QNS. Lorem ipsum dolor sit amet, consectetur adipisicing elit, sed do eiusmod tempor incididunt ut labore et dolore magna aliqua. Ut enim ad minim veniam, quis nostrud exercitation ullamco laboris nisi ut aliquip ex ea commodo consequat. Duis aute irure dolor in reprehenderit in voluptate velit esse cillum dolore eu fugiat nulla pariatur. Excepteur sint occaecat cupidatat non proident, sunt in culpa qui officia deserunt mollit anim id est laborum.

To schedule time with a Personal Health Coach, please call 1-877-4HDLABS (1-877-443-5227) or visit us online at www.myhdl.com

Dr. Joseph P. McConnell | Laboratory Director | CLIA No. 49D1100708 | CAP No. 7224971 | NPI No. 1629209853
©2010 | 737 N. 5th Street Suite 103 | Richmond, Virginia 23219 | Phone: 804.343.2718 | Fax: 804.343.2704

HDL 20.0

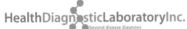

Sterols

Laboratory Test	Notes	Hyper	Optimal	Hypo	Hyper Range	Optimal Range	Hypo Range	Previous Results 9/29/2011
Sterol Absorption Markers								
Campesterol (µg/mL)		7.10			≥ 4.44	2.11 - 4.43	≤ 2.10	
Campesterol Ratio (10² mmol/mol Cholesterol)		245			≥ 241	115 - 240	≤ 114	
Sitosterol (µg/mL)		5.10			≥ 3.18	1.43 - 3.17	≤ 1.42	
Sitosterol Ratio (10² mmol/mol Cholesterol)			141		≥ 169	76 - 168	≤ 75	
Cholestanol (µg/mL)				1.89	≥ 3.48	2.02 - 3.47	≤ 2.01	
Cholestanol Ratio (10² mmol/mol Cholesterol)			145		≥ 195	117 - 194	≤ 116	
Sterol Synthesis Markers								
Desmosterol (µg/mL)		5.10			≥ 1.28	0.50 - 1.27	≤ 0.49	
Desmosterol Ratio (10² mmol/mol Cholesterol)			56		≥ 65	31 - 64	≤ 30	

Lab Notes: Result revised from: 2.3. Result revised from: 1.3. Result revised from: 0.3. QNS. Lorem ipsum dolor sit amet, consectetur adipisicing elit, sed do eiusmod tempor incididunt ut labore et dolore magna aliqua. Ut enim ad minim veniam, quis nostrud exercitation ullamco laboris nisi ut aliquip ex ea commodo consequat. Duis aute irure dolor in reprehenderit in voluptate velit esse cillum dolore eu fugiat nulla pariatur. Excepteur sint occaecat cupidatat non proident, sunt in culpa qui officia deserunt mollit anim id est laborum.

HealthDiagnosticLaboratoryInc.
beyond disease diagnosis

Laboratory Results

Patient

Name: Test M Smith	Phone #: (678) 555-1212	Patient ID #: 12346	
Fasting Status: 12 hours	Gender: Male	Birthdate: 8/12/1928	Age: 83
Height: 5 ft 11 in	Weight: 200 lbs	BMI: 28	Prev. BMI: 9/29/201 28

Specimen

Collection Time: 2:38 pm	Specimen ID: 10022300198
Collection Date: 5/6/2011	Report Type: Complete
Received Date: 5/6/2002	Report Date: 9/29/2011

Provider

Requesting Provider:
Bob Johnson, MD
ABC Family Practice
123 Broad St., Suite 456
Richmond, VA 12345

Client ID:
11-22222-33-4444444

Other Biomarkers	Result	Flag	Reference Interval
Adiponectin (ug/mL)	13		4 - 24
Albumin (g/dl)	3.7		3.5 - 5.2
ALP (U/L)	45		40 - 129
ALT / GPT (U/L)	38		Up to 41
AST / GOT (U/L)	34		Up to 40
BUN (mg/dl)	30		6 - 20
Calcium (mg/dL)	8.7		8.6 - 10.2
CK (U/L)	55		39 - 308
Cl- (mmol/L)	100		96 - 108
CO₂ (mmol/L)	23		22 - 29
D-Dimer (µg/mL)	0.5		< 0.5
Direct Bilirubin (mg/dL)	0.1		0.1 - 0.3
Ester Ratio (%)	74.0		70 - 80%
Ferritin (ng/mL)	389		30 - 400
Free cholesterol (mg/dL)	14.0		
Fructosamine (µmol/L)	208		205 - 285
FSH (mIU/mL)	11.1		1.5 - 12.4
GGT (U/L)	37		8 - 61
Iron (µg/dL)	129		59 - 158
TIBC (µg/dL)	300		250 - 450
K+ (mmol/L)	4.2		3.3 - 5.1
LDH (U/L)	213		< 250
LH (mIU/mL)	7.7		1.7 - 8.6
PSA (ng/mL)	2.0		0.1 - 3.9
Magnesium (mg/dl)	2.30		1.6 - 2.4
Na+ (mmol/L)	142		133 - 145
Phosphorus (mg/dL)	2.9		2.7 - 4.5
Total Bilirubin (mg/dL)	0.8		Up to 1.2
Total Protein (g/dL)	7.3		6.4 - 8.3
T4 (µg/dL)	14.0		4.5 - 11.7
T4, free (ng/dL)	0.96		0.93 - 1.7
T uptake (TBI)	1.2		0.8 - 1.3

CBC with Differential / Platelet	Result	Flag	Units	Reference Interval
WBC	8.9		x10³/µL	4.0 - 10.5
RBC	4.4		x10⁶/µL	4.1 - 5.6
Hemoglobin	15.5		g/dL	12.5 - 17.0
Hematocrit	43		%	36 - 50
MCV	97		fL	80 - 98
MCH	32		pg	27 - 34
MCHC	34		g/dL	32 - 36
RDW	13.0		%	11.7 - 15
Platelets	380		x10³/µL	140 - 415
Neutrophils	73		%	40 - 74
Lymphocytes	45		%	14 - 46
Monocytes	12		%	4 - 13
Eosinophils	6		%	0 - 7
Basophils	2		%	0 - 3
Neutrophils (absolute)	3.5		x10³/µL	1.8 - 7.8
Lymphocytes (absolute)	3.4		x10³/µL	0.7 - 4.5
Monocytes (absolute)	0.9		x10³/µL	0.1 - 1.0
Eosinophils (absolute)	0.2		x10³/µL	0.0 - 0.4
Basophils (absolute)	0.1		x10³/µL	0.0 - 0.2
Immature Granulocytes	0		%	0 - 1
Immature Granulocytes (absolute)	0.1		x10³/µL	0.0 - 0.1

To schedule time with a Personal Health Coach, please call 1-877-4HDLABS (1-877-443-5227) or visit us online at www.myhdi.com

Lab Notes: Result revised from: 2.3. Result revised from: 1.3. Result revised from: 0.3. QNS. Lorem ipsum dolor sit amet, consectetur adipisicing elit, sed do eiusmod tempor incididunt ut labore et dolore magna aliqua. Ut enim ad minim veniam, quis nostrud

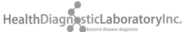

HealthDiagnosticLaboratoryInc.
beyond disease diagnosis

Laboratory Results

Patient

Name:	Phone #:	Patient ID #:
Test M Smith	(678) 555-1212 12346	

Fasting Status:	Gender:	Birthdate:	Age:
12 hours	Male	8/12/1928	83

Height:	Weight:	BMI:	Prev. BMI:
5 ft 11 in	200 lbs	28	9/29/201 28

Specimen

Collection Time:	Specimen ID:
2:38 pm	10022300198

Collection Date:	Report Type:
5/6/2011	Complete

Received Date:	Report Date:
5/6/2002	9/29/2011

Provider

Requesting Provider:
Bob Johnson, MD
ABC Family Practice
123 Broad St., Suite 456
Richmond, VA 12345

Client ID:
11-22222-33-4444444

Other Biomarkers	Result	Flag	Reference Interval
T3 (ng/dL)	94		80 - 200
T3, free (pg/mL)	30.0		> 19 yrs - 2.0 – 4.4
Testosterone (ng/dL)	290		Men: 280 - 800 Boys: < 1 year 12 - 21 1 - 6 years 12 - 32 7 - 12 years 12 - 68 13 - 17 years 28 - 1110

Other	Result	Flag	Reference Interval
β-CrossLaps (pg/mL)	300		30 - 50 years: Mean=300, 1 SD=142, Mean + 2 SD=584 50 - 70 years: Mean=304, 1 SD=200, Mean + 2 SD=704 > 70 years: Mean=394, 1 SD=230, Mean + 2 SD=854
Dehydroepiandrosterone sulfate (µg/dL)	3000		15 - 19 years: 70 - 492 20 - 24 years: 211 - 492 25 - 34 years: 160 - 449 35 - 44 years: 89 - 427 45 - 54 years: 44 - 331 55 - 64 years: 52 - 295 65 - 74 years: 34 - 249 > 75 years: 16 - 123
Estradiol (pg/mL)	32.0		Men: <12 - 42.6 Boys (1-10 Years): <12 - 20
Free Testosterone (ng/dL)	45.20		4.7 - 24.4
Lathosterol (µg/mL)	7.1		0.0 - 7.0
Osteocalcin (ng/mL)	40		7 - 37
Progesterone (ng/mL)	0.76		0.20 - 1.4
PTH, Intact (pg/mL)	8		15 - 65
Human sex hormone-binding globulin (nmol/L)	1000		10 - 80

To schedule time with a Personal Health Coach, please call 1-877-4HDLABS (1-877-443-5227) or visit us online at www.myhdl.com

Lab Notes: Result revised from: 2.3. Result revised from: 1.3. Result revised from: 0.3. QNS. Lorem ipsum dolor sit amet, consectetur adipisicing elit, sed do eiusmod tempor incididunt ut labore et dolore magna aliqua. Ut enim ad minim veniam, quis nostrud exercitation ullamco laboris nisi ut aliquip ex ea commodo consequat. Duis aute irure dolor in reprehenderit in voluptate velit esse cillum dolore eu fugiat nulla pariatur. Excepteur sint occaecat cupidatat non proident, sunt in culpa qui officia deserunt mollit anim id est laborum.

Dr. Joseph P. McConnell | Laboratory Director | CLIA No. 49D1100708 | CAP No. 7224971 | NPI No. 1629209853
©2010 | 737 N. 5th Street Suite 103 | Richmond, Virginia 23219 | Phone: 804.343.2718 | Fax: 804.343.2704

HDL 20.0

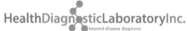

Patient

Name:	Phone #:		Patient ID #:
Test M Smith	(678) 555-1212		12346

Fasting Status:	Gender:	Birthdate:	Age:
12 hours	Male	8/12/1928	83

Height:	Weight:	BMI:	Prev. BMI: 9/29/201
5 ft 11 in	200 lbs	28	28

Specimen

Collection Time:	Specimen ID:
2:38 pm	10022300198

Collection Date:	Report Type:
5/6/2011	Complete

Received Date:	Report Date:
5/6/2002	9/29/2011

Provider

Requesting Provider:
Bob Johnson, MD
ABC Family Practice
123 Broad St., Suite 456
Richmond, VA 12345

Client ID:
11-22222-33-4444444

Lipids

	6/10	6/10	6/10	5/11	9/11	Trend Line	High Risk Range	Intermediate Risk Range	Optimal Range
Total Cholesterol (mg/dL)	220	220	240	29	200		≥ 240	200 - 239	< 200
LDL-C Direct (mg/dL)			90	23	135		≥ 130 CHD & CHD risk eq. > 100	100 - 129 CHD & CHD risk eq. 70 - 100	< 100 CHD & CHD risk eq. < 70
HDL-C (mg/dL)			35	51	70		< 40		≥ 40
Triglycerides (mg/dL)			160		100		≥ 200	150 - 199	< 150

Lipoprotein Particles and Apolipoproteins

	6/10	6/10	6/10	5/11	9/11	Trend Line	High Risk Range	Intermediate Risk Range	Optimal Range
Apo B (mg/dL)				55	85		≥ 80	60 - 79	< 60
LDL-P (nmol/L)			1600	1850	1100		≥ 1300	1000 - 1299	< 1000
HDL2 (mg/dL)*				2	10		≤ 8	9 - 11	≥ 12
Lp(a) Mass (mg/dL)				42	< 12		≥ 30		< 30
Lp(a) Cholesterol (mg/dL)				30	8		≥ 6	3 - 5	< 3

Metabolic

	6/10	6/10	6/10	5/11	9/11	Trend Line	High Risk Range	Intermediate Risk Range	Optimal Range
Insulin (µU/mL)	0				14		≥ 12	10 - 11	3 - 9

HealthDiagnosticLaboratoryInc.
beyond disease diagnosis

Laboratory Results

Patient

Name:	Phone #:	Patient ID #:
Test M Smith	(678) 555-1212	12346

Fasting Status:	Gender:	Birthdate:	Age:
12 hours	Male	8/12/1928	83

Height:	Weight:	BMI:	Prev. BMI:
5 ft 11 in	200 lbs	28	9/29/201 · 28

Specimen

Collection Time:	Specimen ID:
2:38 pm	10022300198

Collection Date:	Report Type:
5/6/2011	Complete

Received Date:	Report Date:
5/6/2002	9/29/2011

Provider

Requesting Provider:
Bob Johnson, MD
ABC Family Practice
123 Broad St., Suite 456
Richmond, VA 12345

Client ID:
11-22222-33-4444444

To schedule time with a Personal Health Coach, please call 1-877-4HDLABS (1-877-443-5227) or visit us online at www.myhdl.com

NMR LipoProfile® Test

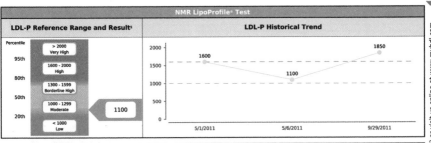

LDL-P Reference Range and Result[1]

Percentile	
95th	> 2000 Very High
80th	1600 - 2000 High
	1300 - 1599 Borderline High
50th	1000 - 1299 Moderate
20th	< 1000 Low

Result: 1100

LDL-P Historical Trend

	5/1/2011	5/6/2011	9/29/2011
	1600	1100	1850

Particle Concentration and Size

	Laboratory Test	Result	Percentile in Reference Population[2]						Previous Results
HDL Particles	**HDL-P (total)** μmol/L	25.0	low	25th (26.7) **25**	50th (30.5)	75th (34.9)		high	

Small LDL-P and LDL Size are associated with CVD risk, but not after LDL-P is taken into account.

	Laboratory Test	Result	Insulin Resistance → Insulin Sensitive						Previous Results
Lipoprotein Markers Associated with Insulin Resistance and Diabetes Risk[4]	**LARGE VLDL-P** nmol/L	0.7	high	75th (6.9)	50th (2.7)	25th (0.9) **0.7**		low	
	SMALL LDL-P nmol/L	70	high	75th (839)	50th (527)	25th (117)	**70**	low	
	LARGE HDL-P μmol/L	2.7	low	25th (3.1) **2.7**	50th (4.8)	75th (7.3)		high	
	VLDL SIZE nm	41.1	large	75th (52.5)	50th (46.6)	25th (42.4) **41.1**		small	45.5
	LDL SIZE nm	20.7	small	25th (20.4)	50th (20.8) **20.7**	75th (21.2)		large	
	HDL SIZE nm	8.5	small **8.5**	25th (8.9)	50th (9.2)	75th (9.6)		large	
	LP-IR SCORE[*] 0 - 100	12	insulin resistant	75th (63)	50th (45)	25th (27)	**12**	insulin sensitive	

LP-IR Score is inaccurate if a patient is non-fasting.
[*]The LP-IR Score combines the information from the 6 markers above it to give improved assessment of insulin resistance and diabetes risk.

These laboratory assays, validated by LipoScience, have not been cleared by the US Food and Drug Administration. The clinical utility of these laboratory values has not been fully established.
1. Reference population comprises '5,362' men and women not on lipid medication enrolled in the Multi-Ethnic Study of Atherosclerosis (MESA). Mora, et al. *Atherosclerosis* 2007.
2. LipoScience reference population comprises 4,588 men and women without known CVD or diabetes and not on lipid medication.
3. Garvey WT, et al. *Diabetes*. 2003; 532:453-462. 4. Goff DC et al. *Metabolism*. 2005; 54:264-270.

Dr. Joseph P. McConnell | Laboratory Director | CLIA No. 49D1100708 | CAP No. 7224971 | NPI No. 1629209853

©2010 | 737 N. 5th Street Suite 103 | Richmond, Virginia 23219 | Phone: 804.343.2718 | Fax: 804.343.2704

HDL 20.0

HealthDiagnosticLaboratoryInc. Omega 3 and Omega 6 Fatty Acids Profile

beyond disease diagnosis

Patient

Name: Test M Smith	Phone #: (678) 555-1212	Patient ID #: 12346
Fasting Status: 12 hours	Gender: Male	Birthdate: 8/12/1928	Age: 83
Height: 5 ft 11 in	Weight: 200 lbs	BMI: 28	Prev. BMI: 9/29/201	28

Specimen

Collection Time: 2:38 pm	Specimen ID: 10022300198
Collection Date: 5/6/2011	Report Type: Complete
Received Date: 5/6/2002	Report Date: 9/29/2011

Provider

Requesting Provider:
Bob Johnson, MD
ABC Family Practice
123 Broad St., Suite 456
Richmond, VA 12345

Client ID:
11-22222-33-4444444

Laboratory Test	Notes	High Risk	Intermediate Risk	Optimal	High Risk Range	Intermediate Risk Range	Optimal Range	Previous Results 9/29/2011
Index HS-Omega-3 Index® (RBC EPA+DHA)ª		3.8			< 4.0%	4.0% - 8.0%	> 8.0%	

Comments:

Your HS-Omega-3 Index is well below the target range of 8%.

The HS-Omega-3 Index is the EPA+DHA content of RBC membranes. Increasing the intake of EPA+DHA by 1 to 2 grams (1,000 - 2,000 mg) per day, from either oily fish or fish oil supplements, should significantly improve the index. The exact amount of EPA+DHA needed will vary person to person. A re-check should be done in 3 - 4 months.

Omega-3 Fatty Acids

Fatty Acids	Range	Current	Previous
Omega-3 Total	0.1% - 14.1%	7.9%	
Alpha-Linolenic (ALA)	0.1% - 0.4%	0.3%	
Docosapentaenoic (DPA)	0.6% - 4.1%	7.4%	
Eicosapentaenoic (EPA)	0.1% - 2.5%	1.2%	
Docosahexaenoic (DHA)	0.1% - 8.4%	4.7%	

Omega-6 Fatty Acids

Fatty Acids	Range	Current	Previous
Omega-6 Total	28.6% - 44.5%	36.9%	
Arachidonic (AA)	10.5% - 23.3%	10.3%	
Linoleic (LA)	4.6% - 21.3%	9.7%	

Other Fatty Acids

Fatty Acids	Range	Current	Previous
cis-Monounsaturated Total	11.5% - 20.5%	12.5%	
Saturated Total	36.6% - 42.0%	40.9%	
Trans Total	<0.1% - 1.8%	2.6%	

Content of EPA+DHA (mg/3 oz serving) in Common Seafoods*

Higher Omega-3	EPA+DHA	Intermediate Omega-3	EPA+DHA	Lower Omega-3	EPA+DHA
Salmon Atlantic, farmed	1825	Swordfish	764	Tuna, Light (canned in water)	230
Herring Atlantic	1712	Rainbow Trout, farmed	744	Halibut	200
Salmon Atlantic	1564	Tuna, Albacore or White (canned in water)	733	Northern Lobster (steamed)	165
Tuna Bluefin	1279	Sockeye Salmon	673	Clams (canned)	150
Salmon Chum	1238	Sea Bass	648	Scallops (steamed)	149
Herring Pickled	1181	Salmon Pink	524	Haddock or Cod	135
Salmon Coho, farmed	1087	Crab Dungeness	501	Mahi-Mahi (dolphin fish)	118
Mackerel (canned)	1046	Alaskan Pollock	433	Tilapia	115
Salmon Coho	900	Crab King	351	Shrimp	87
Oysters (steamed)	850	Walleye	338	Catfish, farmed	76
Sardines (canned in oil)	835	Flat fish (Flounder/sole)	255	Orange Roughy	26

*From the USDA Nutrient Database (as of 8/24/11) for fish cooked with dry heat unless otherwise noted, and wild unless indicated as farmed.

ªThe HS-Omega-3 index cutpoints are based on Harris and von Shacky, Preventive Medicine 2004;39:212-220

To schedule time with a Personal Health Coach, please call 1-877-4HDLABS (1-877-443-5227) or visit us online at www.myhdl.com

Dr. Joseph P. McConnell | Laboratory Director | CLIA No. 49D1100708 | CAP No. 7224971 | NPI No. 1629209853

©2010 | 737 N. 5th Street Suite 103 | Richmond, Virginia 23219 | Phone: 804.343.2718 | Fax: 804.343.2704

HDL 20.0

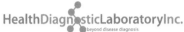

HealthDiagnosticLaboratoryInc.
beyond disease diagnosis

Patient

Name:	Phone #:		Patient ID #:
Test M Smith	(678) 555-1212		12346

Fasting Status:	Gender:	Birthdate:	Age:
12 hours	Male	8/12/1928	83

Height:	Weight:	BMI:	Prev. BMI:
5 ft 11 in	200 lbs	28	28 (9/29/201)

Specimen

Collection Time:	Specimen ID:
2:38 pm	10022300198

Collection Date:	Report Type:
5/6/2011	Complete

Received Date:	Report Date:
5/6/2002	9/29/2011

Provider

Requesting Provider:
Bob Johnson, MD
ABC Family Practice
123 Broad St., Suite 456
Richmond, VA 12345

Client ID:
11-22222-33-4444444

Comments:

Traditional lipoprotein risk factors (total cholesterol and LDL cholesterol) are increased in this sample. Treatment should focus on these abnormalities. Please refer to guidelines from the National Cholesterol Education Program Adult Treatment Panel (ATPIII) for treatment guidelines related to traditional lipid risk factors. Also see: Implications of recent clinical trials for the National Cholesterol Education Program Adult Treatment Panel III Guidelines; Coordinating Committee of the National Cholesterol Education Program. J Am Coll Cardiol. 2004;44:720-32.

Although HDL cholesterol is in the optimal range, large HDL particles (HDL 2) and apolipoprotein A-I are decreased, or in the intermediate range. Low amounts of large HDL particles and apolipoprotein A-I suggest that the HDL present may not be in its most protective form. Large HDL particles (HDL 2) and apolipoprotein A-I concentration may be increased by exercise, fish oil, or alcohol consumption in moderation. Niacin, fibric acids, and combination therapy (statin + niacin) have been demonstrated to increase large HDL particles and Apo A-I.

Small dense LDL cholesterol and Apo B are increased or in the intermediate range, suggesting the presence of small dense LDL particles. Studies have shown that elevated small dense LDL particle concentration is associated with increased risk for coronary heart disease even in the presence of optimal LDL cholesterol values. Small LDL particles may be observed in association with the metabolic syndrome and pre-diabetes. Statin drugs effectively reduce the number of LDL particles, but do not generally influence the size distribution of the LDL particles. Niacin, fibric acids, and combination therapy (statin + niacin) have been shown to increase LDL particle size.

LDL particle concentration is in the intermediate range in this sample. Studies have shown that elevated LDL particle concentration is associated with increased risk for coronary heart disease, even in the presence of optimal LDL cholesterol values. Small LDL particles may be observed in association with the metabolic syndrome and pre-diabetes. Statins effectively reduce the number of LDL particles, but do not generally influence the size distribution of the LDL particles. Niacin, fibrates, and combination therapy (statin +niacin) have been shown to increase LDL particle size.

Increased C-reactive protein. CRP is an acute phase reactant. Data from prospective studies indicates that increased concentration of CRP is associated with an increased risk for the development of ischemic cardiovascular events. Consider repeat analysis of CRP in 2-4 weeks to establish baseline value. If CRP remains elevated, then lifestyle changes, including weight reduction, low-fat diet, smoking cessation and regular exercise, should be the initial approach. A diet rich in plant sterols, soy protein, viscous fiber, and almonds has been shown to have CRP-lowering effects comparable to that of lovastatin 20 mg/day. Medications that may lower CRP include statins, fibrates, aspirin, and fish oil. Reducing global CHD risk by aggressive treatment of the traditional risk factors by established therapies may also be beneficial.

Lp-PLA$_2$ is increased in this sample. Lp-PLA$_2$ is an inflammatory risk marker that, unlike hs-CRP, is not an acute phase reactant. It is produced by macrophages and is a marker of vascular specific inflammation. Lp-PLA$_2$ circulates in the plasma primarily bound to LDL particles. High plasma Lp-PLA$_2$ is associated with increased risk for cardiovascular disease and events (myocardial infarction and stroke). Increased values have also been associated with endothelial dysfunction and peripheral arterial disease. Lp-PLA$_2$ is the only test that is FDA approved to assess risk for stroke. Patients in the upper tertile for both CRP and Lp-PLA$_2$ are at highest risk. In the Atherosclerosis risks in communities (ARIC) study, patients with both CRP and Lp-PLA$_2$ in the upper tertile of the population had 5X increased risk for myocardial infarction and 11X increased risk for stroke. Statins, fibric acids, and niacin have been shown to have Lp-PLA$_2$ lowering effects.

Homocysteine is in the intermediate range. Increases in homocysteine concentration can occur with aging, menopause, hypothyroidism, low plasma levels of vitamin cofactors (B6, B12 and folate), certain drugs, and chronic renal insufficiency. Genetic variation in enzymes involved in homocysteine metabolism contributes to inter-individual differences in plasma homocysteine levels.

Elevated fasting insulin. If a fasting insulin level is elevated, it reflects hyperinsulinemia but fasting levels can be normal when levels following a glucose load are elevated. Insulin is elevated postprandially in proportion to the carbohydrate content in the meal. Elevated fasting insulin levels have been related to atherosclerosis risk. The combination of elevated fasting insulin, apolipoprotein B levels, and small LDL size identifies a very high-risk group for the development of ischemic heart disease.

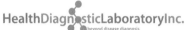

HealthDiagnosticLaboratoryInc.
beyond disease diagnosis

Laboratory Results

Patient

| Name: | Phone #: | Patient ID #: |
| Test M Smith | (678) 555-1212 | 12346 |

| Fasting Status: | Gender: | Birthdate: | Age: |
| 12 hours | Male | 8/12/1928 | 83 |

| Height: | Weight: | BMI: | | Prev. BMI: 9/29/201 | |
| 5 ft 11 in | 200 lbs | 28 | | 28 | |

Specimen

| Collection Time: | Specimen ID: |
| 2:38 pm | 10022300198 |

| Collection Date: | Report Type: |
| 5/6/2011 | Complete |

| Received Date: | Report Date: |
| 5/6/2002 | 9/29/2011 |

Provider

Requesting Provider:
Bob Johnson, MD
ABC Family Practice
123 Broad St., Suite 456
Richmond, VA 12345

Client ID:
11-22222-33-4444444

Comments:

Vitamin D is deficient. Decreased vitamin D has been associated with hypertension, inflammation, and the metabolic syndrome. More recently, low serum 25(OH)D has been associated with increased incidence of cardiovascular events and all cause mortality. One function of vitamin D is to promote calcium absorption in the gut and to maintain adequate blood levels of calcium and phosphorus. If the body does not have adequate supplies of vitamin D, normal bone mineralization is compromised and bones may become thin and brittle. Severe deficiency can lead to rickets, with associate skeletal deformities in children, and osteomalacia in adults, which results in both weak bones and muscles.

The Cystatin C value is elevated in this sample and consequently the estimated glomerular filtration rate (eGFR) is decreased in this patient, which is suggestive of declining kidney function. Cystatin C has been shown to be superior to creatinine for determining an eGFR, and there is a growing body of evidence suggesting that Cystatin C can be used to detect kidney disease at earlier stages than serum creatinine. Recent studies have also demonstrated that increased levels of Cystatin C are associated with an increased risk of heart disease, heart failure, stroke, and mortality. Treatment related to elevated Cystatin C should focus on the underlying kidney disease. Secondary causes of kidney disease, such as diabetes or hypertension should be aggressively treated and managed. Lifestyle changes can be made which may help control kidney disease. The HDL health coaches can help design an eating plan with the correct amounts of sodium, protein and fluid intakes. Routine moderate exercise can also help control kidney function. HDL Health coaches can also help design an exercise program that is right for you.

Apolipoprotein E Genotype is 3/4. In general patients with the E4 allele respond less favorably to pharmacologic therapy with statins. For the ApoE4 allele, simvastatin has evidence of preferred efficacy over other statins, although statins in general are less effective for ApoE4 patients than for patients with 2 or 3 alleles. Subjects with the E4 allele appear to be most responsive to lifestyle changes and are particularly responsive to dietary changes reducing fat and cholesterol intake. Fish oil benefits ApoE2 and E3 patients, but one study demonstrated ApoE4 patients had a 15.9% increase in LDL cholesterol in response to fish oil. This needs to be confirmed in a larger study. ApoE4 patients should follow a healthy diet low in fat and cholesterol and fish oil supplementation should be monitored carefully.

NT-proBNP is in the intermediate range. B-type natriuretic peptide (BNP) is released by the cardiac ventricles in response to increased wall tension and cardiac stress, including cardiac ischemia and inflammation. BNP is synthesized as a prohormone that is cleaved into active BNP and an inactive N-terminal fragment (NT-proBNP). Markedly elevated levels of NT-proBNP are diagnostic of congestive heart failure. Even mildly elevated levels of NT-proBNP lead to an increased risk of future adverse events. In the Ludwigshafen Risk and Cardiovascular Health Study, following 1,135 individuals with and 506 individuals without stable coronary artery disease (CAD) for 5.45 years, NT-pro-BNP concentrations of 100-399, 400-1,999, or >2,000 ng/L resulted in unadjusted hazard ratios (95% CI) for all-cause death of 3.2 (1.8 - 5.6), 6.63 (3.8 - 11.6), and 16.5 (9.2 - 29.8), respectively, compared with concentrations <100 ng/L. Hazard ratios (CI) for death from cardiovascular causes were 3.8 (1.8 - 8.2), 9.3 (4.4 - 19.5), and 22.2 (10.2 - 48.4). Additional clinical information and testing may help determine the etiology of the elevated NT-pro-BNP. Are medications that increase fluid retention (e.g., TZDs) being taken? Does the patient have abnormal ECG (arrhythmias), coronary catheterization, or echo results? Does the patient have renal or pulmonary disorders, or diabetes? Is the patient's blood pressure properly controlled? Repeat analysis of NT-proBNP 1-2 months after specific treatment may be useful to determine the effect of treatment on cardiac function.

The Factor V Leiden genotype for this patient is Arg/Gln, heterozygous carrier. The factor V Leiden mutation has been associated with increased risk for the venous thromboembolism (VTE). Heterozygous carriers of factor V Leiden have an 8 fold increased risk for VTE and homozygous carries have 80 to 100 fold increased risk. For individuals who have previously had a VTE, factor V Leiden carriers are 3 times more likely to have a recurrent DVT than non-carriers, and homozygous carriers are 10-15X more likely to have a recurrence than non-carriers. VTE risk is compounded by concomitant prothrombin G20210A mutations, with compound heterozygotes also having 10-15 fold increased risk of recurrent VTE. More intensive, longer term oral anticoagulant therapy should be considered for factor V Leiden carriers who have previously had a VTE. Carriers who have not previously had a VTE, should take appropriate steps to avoid VTE, such as notify physicians prior to a surgical procedure, and don't sit without moving for long periods of time. Frequently get up, stretch your legs, move around, etc., when on long trips (auto, bus, plane). Women of childbearing age should consider alternative birth control measures than oral contraceptives (OC), as OC use has been associated with increased for VTE and cerebral vein thrombosis in factor V Leiden carriers.

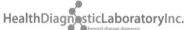

HealthDiagnosticLaboratoryInc.
beyond disease diagnosis

Laboratory Results

Patient

Name:	Phone #:	Patient ID #:
Test M Smith	(678) 555-1212	12346

Fasting Status:	Gender:	Birthdate:	Age:
12 hours	Male	8/12/1928	83

Height:	Weight:	BMI:	Prev. BMI: 9/29/201
5 ft 11 in	200 lbs	28	28

Specimen

Collection Time:	Specimen ID:
2:38 pm	10022300198

Collection Date:	Report Type:
5/6/2011	Complete

Received Date:	Report Date:
5/6/2002	9/29/2011

Provider

Requesting Provider:
Bob Johnson, MD
ABC Family Practice
123 Broad St., Suite 456
Richmond, VA 12345

Client ID:
11-22222-33-4444444

Comments:

This patient is homozygous (T/T) for the methylenetetrahydrofolate reductase (MTHFR) polymorphism. This indicates that this patient's enzyme is thermolabile and does not effectively metabolize folic acid (folate). Methylfolate is the active form of folate. Patients with homozygosity for this polymorphism are more likely to have elevated homocysteine values. Patients with high homocysteine values who are homozygous for the MTHFR polymorphism will not respond as well to folate supplementation with folic acid and consideration should be given to supplementation with the active methylfolate. Although homocysteine is an independent risk factor for cardiovascular disease and events, treatment of elevated homocysteine with folic acid and B vitamins (B6 and B12) has not been shown to decrease events. Consideration should be given to more aggressive treatment of other CV risk factors in patients with elevated homocysteine. Other homocysteine lowering efforts which may be beneficial include methyl folate and/or betaine supplementation.

Total HDL particle concentration is decreased in this sample. Decreased HDL particles have been associated with increased risk for cardiovascular disease. HDL particle concentration may be increased by exercise, fish oil, or alcohol consumption in moderation. Niacin, fibric acids, and combination therapy (statin + niacin) have been demonstrated to increase HDL particle concentration.

This patient is heterozygous for the CYP2C9*3 allele, homozygous for the VKORC1 allele and has the normal or wild type genotype for the CYP2C9*2 allele. Patients who have these mutations have a decreased ability to metabolize the drug warfarin. Patients with these mutations are predisposed to warfarin sensitivity and require lower doses of warfarin to reach the desired International Normalized Ratio (INR).

An algorithm for estimating warfarin dose, based on multi-regression models including age, gender, height, weight, genotype, multidrug interactions, INR, and other characteristics, is available at www.warfarindosing.org. Genotype information can be incorporated into estimating the starting dose of warfarin and may also impact adjustments until stable dosing is achieved.

No other CYP2C9 and VKORC1 variants, other than those listed, were tested for.

Results for the Adiponectin test are for research purposes only by the assay's manufacturer. The performance characteristics of this product have not been established. Results should not be used as a diagnostic procedure without confirmation of the diagnosis by another medically established diagnostic product or procedure.

End of Report

ATTN PATIENT: Please contact HDL, Inc. at 1-877-4HDLABS (1-877-443-5227) to set an appointment with your personal health coach to discuss your diet and exercise needs at no charge. You can also visit us online at www.myhdl.com and schedule an appointment through our web portal.

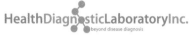
HealthDiagnosticLaboratoryInc.
beyond disease diagnosis

Warfarin Dosing

Venous thromboembolism (VTE) is a syndrome whereby thrombosis (a blood clot) occurs in the deep veins and which may result in a Pulmonary Embolism (PE). Both genetic and environmental factors may predispose an individual to VTE. Physicians may order testing for warfarin dosing in individuals diagnosed with, or genetically predisposed to, VTE, so that optimal warfarin loading and maintenance doses can be determined.

A Deep Vein Thrombosis (DVT) is a blood clot in a vein deep below the surface of the skin, usually occurring in the legs. A Pulmonary Embolism occurs when a DVT breaks loose and travels to the lungs. A PE is a potentially fatal condition and the reason DVT is so concerning in the first place. DVT can happen either spontaneously or after surgery. DVT is more likely to happen due to a lack of movement and is most common when stuck in bed or on a plane for long periods.

DVT can also be associated with injury – even minor ones.

Symptoms of DVT:

- Swelling, pain or tenderness in a leg, which may only be felt when standing or walking.
- Increased warmth, redness or purple coloring on the skin near the swelling.

Symptoms of PE:

- Unexplained shortness of breath.
- Rapid breathing and fast heart rate (pulse).
- Pain when taking a deep breath.
- Coughing up blood.

Unfortunately, sometimes the first indication of a DVT is when it develops into a PE.

To lower your risk and help prevent DVT, try to maintain an active lifestyle and exercise regularly - daily if possible. Walking, swimming and cycling are all excellent activities. The back of the attached Medical Information Card provides tips for preventing DVT and PE.

To remove card, fold along perforated lines and cut with scissors or tear gently.

MEDICAL INFORMATION

Name: Test M Smith

Your physician ordered this testing for warfarin dosing because you have had Venous thromboembolism (VTE), or may be at increased risk for VTE because of genetic or other causes. This card provides your warfarin dosing genotypes for 3 variants that will assist your medical caregiver in the event you require warfarin anticoagulation.

CYP2C9*2: C/C CYP2C9*3: C/A VKORC1: A/A

Your caregiver should visit **www.warfarindosing.org** to calculate appropriate dosing.
Please see reverse of card for tips to avoid DVT. Patient ID: 12346

MEDICAL INFORMATION

To lower your risks and help prevent DVT, take these 5 simple steps.

1. Maintain good circulation.
   - Establish an active lifestyle with regular exercise.
   - Prevent DVT when traveling.
     ✓ Drink plenty of fluids. Avoid dehydrating fluids (e.g., coffee and alcohol).
     ✓ Avoid short, tight stockings.
     ✓ Avoid crossing legs for long periods of time.
     ✓ When traveling by car, stop every hour and walk around.
     ✓ When traveling by plane, get up and move around at least once an hour.
2. For birth control, consider alternatives to oral contraceptives.
3. In pregnancy, notify obstetrician of genetic predisposition to VTE prior to delivery.
4. Notify surgeon / physician of predisposition and the need for an appropriate anticoagulant during ANY surgical procedure.
5. Control homocysteine and fibrinogen levels.

There has been a monumental shift in the scientific understanding of the role of cholesterol in metabolic disorders and coronary heart disease (CHD). Various labs offer custom panels of tests beyond the conventional lipid panel. Physicians can personalize treatment based on a comprehensive patient profile including a number of cholesterol components, advanced risk factors, genetic and other biomarkers. This approach allows earlier detection of disease, more targeted treatments, and ultimately fewer heart attacks, strokes, and vascular events.

Diseases of the heart and vascular system remain the major cause of morbidity and mortality in the developed world and are rapidly overtaking other diseases in developing countries. National and international guidelines for intervention have focused on LDL, the major carrier of cholesterol in the circulation. The association of cholesterol with coronary heart disease has long been recognized, as evidenced by the early 1900s experimental production of atherosclerosis in rabbits fed a diet high in cholesterol.

Cholesterol, even though an essential element of cell membranes and precursor to the necessary steroid hormones and vitamin D, has engendered a negative or pathological connotation; e.g., its presence was first recognized and measured in gallstones followed by the association with atherosclerosis and cardiovascular disease.

When the lipoprotein carriers were first recognized in the mid-1900s, it must have seemed logical to measure LDL and the other lipoproteins in terms of their cholesterol content, because assays existed for cholesterol, which were subsequently adapted for serum assays. Hence, the many subsequent epidemiology and intervention studies focused on LDL-cholesterol as the primary atherogenic risk factor. Mainstream practice today continues to follow this precedent.

Nevertheless, subsequent studies have shown clearly that the protein constituents, e.g., Apolipoprotein B (ApoB), the major protein of LDL, and ApoA-I, the major protein of the primarily protective HDL fraction, are better indicators of risk association and response to treatment. Furthermore, it is now recognized that each of the major lipoprotein classes is heterogenous, with a variety of sub-particle classes and other constituents, characterization of which can improve the estimation of CVD risk.

Other contributors to cardiovascular disease, such as metabolic disorders and consequent inflammation, have been recognized as contributing to disease progression. This developing awareness provides the foundation for advanced testing of cardiovascular risk factors and biomarkers. Such advanced tests can substantially clarify contributors to cardiovascular disease and improve management of patients.

Mainstream treatment guidelines focus on the statin class of cholesterol-lowering drugs, which have been proven in many studies to be effective in decreasing incidence of various manifestations of cardiovascular disease. The statins have become the standard of care and are widely prescribed and increasingly more effective. Nevertheless, even high-dose therapies with the newer, most effective statins leave a residual risk. Some patients will continue to progress and suffer events in spite of apparently effective treatment.

Statins tend to lower cholesterol across the range of LDL particles and may leave substantial amounts of the more atherogenic small, dense LDL particles. Combination therapies with niacin, fibrates, and other compounds may have differential and additive effect in further relieving the residual risk.

Elevated LDL-C/ApoB/LDL-P

Disorder

Elevated LDL-C
- An independent risk factor for CVD
- NCEP-ATP III guidelines' primary target is LDL-C lowering

Elevated ApoB
- ApoB is the scientifically accepted measurement of atherogenic particle number. ApoB traverses in the blood in a 1:1 ratio with chylomicrons, VLDL, IDL, LDL and Lp(a)
- Several studies identified elevated ApoB concentrations to be highly predictive of cardiovascular events
- Most studies found ApoB to be a more reliable indicator of cardiovascular event risk than LDL-C

Elevated LDL-P
- Determined by NMR (Nuclear Magnetic Resonance)
- Best utilized in high-risk CVD patients
- Elevated LDL particle concentration associated with increased CHD risk even with optimal LDL-C

Relative Risk

2–3 X increased risk of CVD

Causative Factors

Hereditary Component
Lifestyle
- High fat intake
- Sedentary routine

Conditions
- Overweight/obesity
- Diabetes
- Hypothyroidism
- Renal dysfunction
- Cystic fibrosis

Therapeutic Options

Lifestyle
- Dietary restrictions
- Exercise accompanied by reduction in dietary fat intake
- Weight loss (as appropriate)

Medications
- Statins
- Niacin
- Resins (BAS)
- Fenofibrate
- Niacin + statin combination
- Statin + fenofibrate combination
- Zetia® (ezetemibe)

Therapeutic Goal

LDL-C
  < 100 mg/dL
  < 70 mg/dL with CHD & CHD Risk Equivalents

ApoB
  ≤ 60 mg/dL
  < 55 mg/dL with CHD & CHD Risk Equivalents

LDL-P
  < 1000 nmol/L

Elevated Small Dense LDL Particles (sdLDL)/% sdLDL

Disorder

Elevated sdLDL
- Associated with atherogenic lipoprotein profile with high triglycerides & low HDL-C
- In patients with CHD, 50% of men & 30% of women typically have sdLDL
- Small size enhances endothelial penetration & accelerates atherosclerosis and lipoprotein oxidation
- Commonly present in insulin resistant patients

Elevated % sdLDL
- Calculated value
- sdLDL/direct LDL-C X 100 = % sdLDL
- Greater emphasis should be placed on sdLDL vs. % sdLDL

Relative Risk

3 X increased risk of MI & stroke

Causative Factors

Hereditary Component
Lifestyle
- High fat intake
- Sedentary routine

Conditions
- Overweight/obesity
- Smoking
- Insulin resistance
- Diabetes mellitus
- Cardiometabolic disease

Therapeutic Options

Lifestyle
- Dietary restrictions
- Exercise
- Weight loss (as appropriate)
- Smoking cessation
- Moderate alcohol intake (dependent on ApoE genotype)
- Treat diabetes mellitus & insulin resistance

Medications
- Niacin
- Fenofibrate

- Statins (reduce concentration of sdLDL particles, but do not change particle size)
- Pioglitazone
- Fish oil

Therapeutic Goal

sdLDL
  ≤ 20 mg/dL
  % sdLDL
  ≤ 13%

Low HDL-C

Disorder

- An independent risk factor for CVD
- Major class of lipoproteins responsible for reverse cholesterol transport
- A secondary goal of NCEP ATP III
- Inversely associated with CVD
- For every 1% decrease in HDL-C levels, the risk of a coronary event is thought to increase by 2%
- Low levels of HDL-C increase cardiovascular risk whether LDL-C is low, average or high
- Functionality of HDL-C affects outcomes and ongoing work is being done to better understand HDL-C functionality

Relative Risk

2.5 X increased risk of CVD (If HDL-C<35mg/dL & TCHOL<200 mg/dL)
5 X increased risk of CVD (If HDL-C<35 mg/dL & TCHOL 200–300 mg/dL)

Causative Factors

Hereditary Component
Lifestyle
  - High consumption of dietary fats (dependent on ApoE genotype)
  - High cabohydrate intake
  - Sedentary routine
  - Smoking
Conditions
  - Increasing age
  - Overweight/obesity
  - Insulin resistance
  - Uncontrolled type 2 diabetes mellitus
  - Consistency with diabetes

- Liver & kidney dysfunction
- Hyperthyroidism
- High CETP or hepatic lipase activity

Therapeutic Options

Lifestyle
- Fat restricted cardio-protective diet (dependent on ApoE genotype)
- Walnuts/almonds & flaxseed
- Weight loss (as appropriate)
- Aerobic exercise
- Moderate alcohol intake (dependent on ApoE genotype)
- Smoking cessation
- Treat diabetes mellitus & insulin resistance

Medications
- Niacin
- Niacin + statin
- Fenofibrate
- Statin + fenofibrate
- Pioglitazone
- Fish oil—dependent on ApoE genotype

Therapeutic Goal

NCEP ATP III Goal
Men & Women
$\geq 40mg/dL$
HDL, Inc. Goal
Women
≥ 50 mg/dL
Men
≥ 40 mg/dL

Low ApoA-I

Disorder
- Major proteins found in HDL-C and TRIG-rich lipoproteins
- Low levels are associated with low levels of HDL-C and reduced cholesterol clearance
- Most useful in characterizing patients with genetic disorders

Relative Risk
3 X increased risk of MI and stroke

Causative Factors

Hereditary Component
Lifestyle
- High consumption of dietary fats (dependent on ApoE genotype)
- Smoking

Conditions
- Uncontrolled diabetes
- Chronic renal failure
- Acute hepatitis
- Cirrhosis

Therapeutic Options

Lifestyle
- Exercise
- Weight loss (as appropriate)
- Low fat diet

Medications
- Niacin
- Statins
- Fenofibrate
- Estrogen
- Pioglitazone

Therapeutic Goal
Women
≥ 151 mg/dL
Men
≥ 132 mg/dL

Low HDL2

Disorder

- HDL subclass associated with the majority of reverse cholesterol transport
- Possibly a marker for plaque regression
- Thought to have anti-oxidant properties

Relative Risk

2–3 X increased risk of CVD

Causative Factors

Hereditary Component

Lifestyle
- High fat diet (dependent on ApoE genotype)
- High carbohydrate intake
- Sedentary routine (dependent on ApoE genotype)
- Smoking

Conditions
- Increasing age
- High triglycerides
- Overweight/obesity
- Insulin resistance
- Diabetes mellitus
- Liver, kidney & thyroid disease

Therapeutic Options

Lifestyle
- Fat restricted cardio-protective diet (dependent on ApoE genotype)
- Aerobic exercise
- Weight loss (as appropriate)
- Smoking cessation
- Treat diabetes mellitus & insulin resistance

Medications
- Niacin
- Niacin + statin
- Fish oil—dependent on ApoE genotype

Therapeutic Goal

Women
  ≥ 17 mg/dL
Men
  ≥ 12 mg/dL

Elevated ApoB:ApoAI Ratio

Disorder

- Calculated value
  ApoB/ApoA-I = ApoB:ApoA-I ratio
- Better than traditional cholesterol measures and ratios for estimating MI risk (INTERHEART & AMORIS studies)

Relative Risk

3 X increased risk of MI and stroke

Causative Factors

**See causative factors for elevated ApoB and elevated ApoA-I

Therapeutic Options

- Aggressively lower ApoB and raise ApoA-I with previously suggested therapeutic options

Therapeutic Goal

≤ 0.6

Elevated Triglycerides

Disorder

- An atherogenic characteristic of the metabolic syndrome
- Hypertriglyceridemia a secondary goal in NCEP ATP III guidelines
- VLDL usually contain large quantities of triglycerides
- Hypertriglyceridemia associates with high levels of remnant lipoproteins and vascular inflammatory factors
- Levels >500mg/dL should be treated aggressively to prevent acute pancreatitis

Relative Risk

2–3 X increased risk of CVD

Causative Factors

Hereditary Component
Lifestyle
- High carbohydrate intake
- Fat intake
- Sedentary routine
- Smoking Conditions
- Overweight/obesity
- Hypothyroidism
- Insulin resistance
- Diabetes mellitus
- Alcoholism
- Renal dysfunction
- Pregnancy Medications
- Anabolic steroids
- Oral contraceptives
- Non-selective beta blockers

- Thiazide diuretics
- Corticosteroids
- Some HIV drugs

Therapeutic Options

Lifestyle
- Reduce fat intake (dependent on ApoE genotype)
- Avoid high carbohydrate diet
- Exercise
- Weight loss (as appropriate)
- Avoid alcohol intake

Medications
- Niacin
- Niacin + statin combination
- Fenofibrate
- Fish oil
- Pioglitazone
- Statins

NCEP ATP III Goal

< 150 mg/dL
< 90 mg/dL
correlates with control of insulin resistance and improved cardiovascular outcomes

Elevated Lp(a) Mass/Lp(a) Cholesterol

Disorder

Lp(a) Mass
- An LDL particle containing an abnormal protein
- Inherited abnormality
- High levels associated with an increased risk of developing coronary artery disease
- Levels commonly three times higher in African American population vs. Asian, Oceanic, or European populations
- Structure similar to plasminogen; competes with plasminogen for receptor sites, causing reduced fibrinolysis and increased hypercoagulability

Lp(a) Cholesterol
- When Lp(a) mass ≥30mg/dL, HDL, Inc. reflexes to measure Lp(a) cholesterol
- This reflex eliminates false positives that result from the Lp(a) mass immunoassay

- Such false positives are due to overestimation of large species with high number of kringle repeats

Relative Risk

3–5 X increased risk of CVD

Causative Factors

Hereditary Component
Lifestyle
- Has no impact on Lp(a) mass or Lp(a) cholesterol
Conditions
- Renal disease
- Familial hypercholesterolemia
- Uncontrolled diabetes mellitus
- Low estrogen levels (postmenopause)

Therapeutic Options

Lifestyle
- Treat all other lipoprotein disorders aggressively
Medications
- Niacin
- Estrogen (risk/benefit decision)
- Fenofibrate (limited efficacy)
- Aspirin
- Some statins may elevate Lp(a) mass in patients

Therapeutic Goal

Lp(a) mass
  < 30 mg/dL
Lp(a) chol
  < 2 mg/dL

ApoE Genotype

ApoE is produced primarily in the liver and brain. ApoE containing lipoproteins transport lipids obtained from the diet to the tissues for storage, and from the tissues to the liver for excretion.

ApoE4 (3/4, 4/4, 2/4) Estimated Frequency in Humans: 3/4 ≈25%, 4/4 ≈1-2%, 2/4 ≈1-2%

Inherited Trait

Associations
- High risk for CVD
- Increased triglycerides
- Increased TC, LDL-C
- Lower HDL-C and HDL2-C
- Most importantly increased ApoB and LDL-P
- More severe coronary lesions
- Alzheimer's syndrome
- Increased risk from smoking

Testing Recommendations
- Omega-3 & Omega-6 Fatty Acid Profile
- Non-cholesterol Sterols/Stanols (markers of cholesterol absorption and synthesis)
- Insulin resistance markers

Therapeutic Options

Lifestyle
- Very low-saturated fat diet and no trans fats
- No refined carbohydrates
- Smoking cessation
- Daily physical exercise
- Diet with plenty of fresh fruit and vegetables
- Soluble fiber
- Omega-3 supplementation to normalize omega-3 index

Medications
- LDL receptor therapies (statins, ezetimibe, bile acid sequestrants) and follow sterol absorption markers
- Fenofibrate and niacin as needed
- Follow LDL-P and ApoB in addition to lipid levels

ApoE2 (2/2 & 2/3) Estimated Frequency in Humans: 2/2 ≈1-2%, 2/3 ≈15%

Inherited Trait

Associations (general)
- In general lower CV risk
- Decreased TC, LDL-C, and ApoB

Associations with Type III Familial Dysbetalipoproteinemia (E2/2)
- Hypothyroidism
- PCOS, Diabetes, Lipodystrophy
- Obesity
- Increased triglycerides
- Increased VLDL-P
- TG-raising effect of some medications
- Increased IDL-P
- Significant increases in TC, LDL-C, and TG with unremarkable LDL-P and ApoB

Therapeutic Options
(for E2/E2 and Type III)

Lifestyle
- Avoid obesity
- Maintain insulin sensitivity
- Moderate-fat diet (≤35% fat) – low in saturated fat, no trans fats
- No refined carbohydrates
- Regular physical exercise
- Smoking cessation
- Diet with plenty of fresh fruit and vegetables
- Omega-3 supplementation to normalize omega-3 index

Medications (Type III)
- Statin/fibrate combination
- High dose fish oils if needed to decrease TG
- Other meds as needed to get to goal (e.g., BA sequestrants, plant stanol)

ApoE3 (3/3) Estimated Frequency in Humans: 3/3 ≈55%

Inherited Trait

Associations
- Considered 'wildtype' (or normal) lipid metabolism

Therapeutic Options
(if dislipidemia present)

Lifestyle
- Diet low in saturated fat and no trans fats
- No refined carbohydrates
- Soluble fiber

- Regular physical exercise
- Smoking cessation
- Omega-3 supplementation to normalize omega-3 index

Medications
- Statins
- Statin/ezetimibe
- Plant stanol (Benecol)

Elevated Lp-PLA2

Disorder

- Lipoprotein-associated phospholipase A2; aka plateletactivating factor acetylhydrolase (PAF-AH) is an enzyme associated with atherosclerotic lesions and primarily carried on LDL and Lp(a) in the circulation
- An indicator of arterial inflammation that has been associated with increased risk of CAD and especially high risk for ischemic stroke
- A risk factor for CVD independent of LDL-C
- High levels found in circulation when vulnerable, inflamed, rupture-prone plaque are present
- Cleaves oxidized LDL-C in endothelium, & attracts inflammatory cells (macrophages)
- Macrophages then engulf LDL-C particles forming foam cells
- Lp-PLA2 activity correlates with coronary calcification

Relative Risk

2 X increased risk of CVD
5.5 X increased risk of stroke
11.4 X increased risk of stroke when hs-CRP & Lp-PLA2 are elevated
6.4 X increased risk of stroke when systolic BP is elevated

Causative Factors

Lifestyle
- Smoking

Conditions
- Low HDL-C
- Familial hypercholesterolemia
- Obstructive sleep apnea
- Untreated or ineffectively treated depression/anxiety/bipolar/ mental health disorders

- Thyroid disorders
- Hypertension
- Autoimmune disorders
- Chronic kidney disease
- Dyslipidemia

Therapeutic Options

Lifestyle
- Diet
- Exercise

Medications
- Statins
- Niacin
- Fenofibrate
- Fish oil
- Statin + niacin + fish oils combination
- Ezetimibe
- Aspirin (325mg) for anti-platelet benefits if vulnerable lesion ruptures

Therapeutic Goal

< 200 ng/mL

Elevated High-sensitivity C-reactive Protein (hs-CRP)

Disorder

- CRP is a non-specific acute phase reactant produced by the liver in response to any inflammatory process elsewhere in the body. The test for hs-CRP refers to a high sensitivity assay capable of detecting low levels of CRP associated with vascular inflammation
- Many studies suggest that after adjusting for other factors, hs-CRP is useful as a risk predictor
- High levels of hs-CRP consistently predict recurrent coronary events in patients with unstable angina & acute myocardial infarction
- Higher hs-CRP levels also associated with lower survival rates in these patients
- hs-CRP 2.0 mg/L regardless of LDL-C level is associated with increased CVD risk, and is a useful test for identifying higher risk individuals (JUPITER study)

Relative Risk

2–3 X increased risk of CVD

Causative Factors

Lifestyle
- Smoking
- Stress
- Sedentary routine

Conditions
- Inflammatory conditions
- Infection
- Rheumatoid arthritis
- Cardiovascular disorders
- Hypertension
- Angina
- MI
- Metabolic disorders
- Insulin resistance
- Hyperglycemia
- Overweight/obesity

Medications
- Oral contraceptives

Therapeutic Options

Lifestyle
- Diet rich in plant sterols, soy protein, viscous fiber & almonds
- Exercise
- Smoking cessation
- Weight loss (as appropriate)

Medications
- Statins
- Fenofibrate
- Pioglitazone
- Aspirin (325mg)
- Niacin
- ACE Inhibitors
- Angiotensin receptor blockers
- Metformin
- Beta blockers
- Platelet aggregation inhibitors

Therapeutic Goal

< 1 mg/L

Elevated Fibrinogen

Disorder

- Fibrinogen is a protein that converts to fibrin in forming blood clots and is also an acute phase reactant, responding to any inflammatory process including atherosclerotic lesions in the arteries
- Elevated fibrinogen has been shown to associate with increased risk for CVD, especially in the presence of elevated atherogenic lipoproteins
- HDL, Inc. determines fibrinogen mass rather than the more common fibrinogen activity assay
- Involved in coagulation cascade; increases blood viscosity & platelet aggregation
- Elevated levels enhance platelet adhesion & can cause a prothrombotic state
- Increased levels increase the risk of stroke independent of other cardiovascular risk factors

Relative Risk

2–3 X increased risk of CVD

Causative Factors

Hereditary Component
Lifestyle
- Smoking
- Sedentary routine
- Stress (especially in men)

Conditions
- Advancing age
- Post-menopausal females
- Overweight/obesity
- Diabetes mellitus
- Insulin resistance
- Inflammation
- Hyperlipidemia
- Hypertension

Medications
- Oral contraceptives
- Gemfibrozil

Therapeutic Options

Lifestyle

- Weight loss (as appropriate)
- Smoking cessation
- Exercise
- Moderate alcohol intake (dependent on ApoE genotype)

Medications
- Niacin
- Fenofibrate
- Aspirin
- Fish oil
- Atorvastatin
- Simvastatin

Therapeutic Goal

$\leq$ 390 mg/dL

Elevated Homocysteine

Disorder

- Homocysteine is an amino acid intermediate in methionine and cysteine metabolism. As Vitamin B12 and folic acid are required for conversion, elevated homocysteine can signal deficiencies in these vitamins. Homocysteine is often a by-product when your body digests protein
- High levels cause endothelial dysfunction, vascular injury, smooth muscle proliferation, & thrombogenicity
- Augments the production of oxidized LDL-C
- Commonly used as a screen for patients at risk for CVD & stroke, especially if there are no other risk factors except family history

Relative Risk

2–3 X increased risk of CVD

Causative Factors

Hereditary Metabolic Defects
Lifestyle
- High meat intake
- Low green vegetable intake
- High alcohol ingestion
- High caffeine intake
- Nicotine use (cigarettes, pipe, cigar, tobacco chewing)

Conditions
- Advancing age

- Folic acid, vitamins B6 & B12 deficiencies
- Hypothyroidism
- Leukemia
- Renal dysfunction
- Pernicious anemia
- Post-menopausal females

Medications
- Niacin
- Fenofibrate
- Methotrexate
- Anticonvulsants
- Cholestyramine
- Metformin
- Cyclosporin

Therapeutic Options

Lifestyle
- Diet including green leafy vegetables

Treat existing conditions
- Renal dysfunction
- Pernicious anemia
- Hypothyroidism

Medications
- Controversial as trials to date have been inconclusive regarding the initiation and effect of folic acid, vitamin B6 & vitamin B12 supplementation

Therapeutic Goal

≤ 10 µmol/L

Elevated NT-proBNP

Disorder

- N-terminal pro B type natriuretic peptide (NT-proBNP) is co-secreted with BNP by the ventricles of the heart in response to excessive stretching of heart muscle cells (cardiomyocytes)
- Independent predictor of cardiovascular mortality and other cardiac composite endpoints in patients with risk of CAD, diagnosed CAD, and diagnosed HF
- Provides assessment of left ventricular systolic & diastolic dysfunction
- A useful indicator for even mild heart failure
- Can help distinguish the difference between pulmonary and cardiac

causes of shortness of breath
- Used for screening and diagnosis of congestive heart failure as well as to determine prognosis and risk for adverse events

Relative Risk

3.8 X increased risk of CVD (if NT-proBNP is 100–399 pg/mL)
9.3 X increased risk of CVD (if NT-proBNP is 400–1999 pg/mL)
22 X increased risk of death from CV causes (if NT-proBNP is >2000 pg/mL)

Causative Factors

Conditions
- Advancing age
- Heart failure
- Cardiomyopathy
- Hypertension
- Myocardial infarction
- Dysrhythmias
- Diabetes mellitus
- Pulmonary conditions
  - COPD
  - Pulmonary embolism
- Sepsis
- Renal dysfunction
- Diastolic dysfunction
- ACS

Therapeutic Options

Medications
- Selection depends on cause of cardiac dysfunction
- Preload reducing agents (diuretics, nitrates)
- Afterload reducing agents (ACE inhibitors, ARBs, calcium channel blockers & alpha blockers)
- In patients with diastolic dysfunction, adequate heart rate control with a calcium channel blocker or betablocker is recommended to prevent sudden bouts of tachycardia, which may result in flash pulmonary edema
- Additional interventions may include:
  - Surgery
  - Percutaneous coronary intervention
  - Cardiac ablation
  - Cardiac pacing
- Ranolazine (late phase sodium current inhibitor)

Therapeutic Goal

< 125 pg/mL for patients < 75 years of age
< 450 pg/mL for patients > 75 years of age

Elevated Insulin

Disorder

- Insulin is a hormone produced by the beta cells of the pancreas, which is responsible for regulating blood levels of glucose by facilitating uptake of glucose by cells for energy or for storage
- Progressive elevated insulin levels are significantly associated with insulin resistance as well as atherosclerosis & CVD risk
- Upper Tertile ≥ 12.4 µU/mL

Relative Risk

6 X increased risk for ischemic heart disease, insulin resistance, metabolic syndrome & diabetes

Causative Factors

Hereditary Component
Lifestyle
- Sedentary routine
- Stress
- High carbohydrate diet

Conditions
- Advancing age
- Drop in estrogen levels (post-menopause)
- Non-caucasian ancestry
- Obesity (esp. with visceral adiposity)
- Chronic inflammation
- Insulin resistance
- Type-2 diabetes mellitus
- Metabolic syndrome
- Cushing's syndrome
- Polycystic ovarian syndrome
- Hemochromatosis
- Elevations may extraneously be caused by:
  - Postprandial blood sample
  - Exogenous administration of regular insulin
  - Corticosteroids

Therapeutic Options

Lifestyle
- Fat-restricted cardio-protective diet
- Limit carbohydrates
- Utilize high fiber
- Weight loss (as appropriate)
- Regular exercise (aerobic & weight training)

Medications
- Metformin
- TZDs
- Incretin mimetics
- DPP4 inhibitors
- Basal insulin
- Glipizide/glyburide
- Alpha-glucosidase inhibitors (Acarbose)
- Fenofibrate

Therapeutic Goal

3–9 µU/mL

Elevated Free Fatty Acids/Non-Esterified Fatty Acids (FFA/NEFA)

Disorder

- Fatty acids not attached to triglycerides or phospholipids are called free fatty acids. Elevated FFA/NEFA is associated with insulin resistance, metabolic syndrome & type-2 diabetes
- FFA's activate inflammatory processes involved in atherogenic plaque
- Increased plasma free fatty acids induce markers of endothelial function, vascular inflammation, and thrombosis
- Impairs insulin action in skeletal muscle
- Stimulates VLDL and TRIG production and lowers HDL-C production
- Increased vasoconstriction and Na+ reabsorption
- Blocks glucose uptake by tissues including muscle, liver, and betacells of the pancreas, contributing to elevated blood glucose

Relative Risk

1.6 X increased risk of hypertension
Increases risk of raising glucose levels
Increases risk for beta cell death by lipotoxicity

Causative Factors

Lifestyle
- Sedentary
- Prolonged fasting/starvation

Conditions
- Obesity
- Diabetes
- Metabolic syndrome
- Endocrinopathies
  - Pheochromocytoma
  - Glucagon, thyrotropin, and adrenocorticotropin secreting tumors

Therapeutic Options

Lifestyle
- Weight loss (as appropriate)
- Exercise
- Low carbohydrate diet

Medications
- Niacin
- Fenofibrate
- Pioglitazone/Rosiglitazone
- Glucophage® (metformin)
- Pioglitazone/Rosiglitazone & metformin combination

Therapeutic Goal

≤ 0.59 mmol/L

Low 25-Hydroxy-Vitamin D

Disorder
- Vitamin D deficiency defined as 25-hydroxy-vitamin D level <20 ng/mL
- Vitamin D insufficiency defined as 25-hydroxy-vitamin D level of 20 to 30 ng/mL
- Deficiency of 25-hydroxy-vitamin D associated with:
  - atherosclerosis
  - up-regulation of renin-angiotensin-aldosterone system
  - hypertension
  - insulin resistance
  - diabetes mellitus
  - metabolic syndrome

- hypocalcemia & hypophosphatemia
- Associated with increased incidence of cardiovascular events, cancer, osteoperosis & all cause mortality

Relative Risk

2 X increased risk of CVD (if <10ng/mL)

Causative Factors

Lifestyle
- Age: elderly & newborns
- Inadequate sun exposure
- Homebound
- Increased distance from equator
- Winter season
- Cover-up clothing
- Sunscreen
- Environment
- Air pollution

Conditions
- Obesity
- Malabsorption
- Renal dysfunction
- Liver dysfunction

Therapeutic Options

Lifestyle
- Sun exposure
- High vitamin D diet

Medications
- Vitamin D3 (cholecalciferol)
- Vitamin D2 (ergocalciferol)
- Vitamin D-fortified milk

Therapeutic Goal

30–100 ng/mL

Elevated Myeloperoxidase (MPO)

Disorder

- Myeloperoxidase is an enzyme synthesized and stored within polymorphonuclear leukocytes (PMNs) and monocytes.

- MPO reduces bioavailability of nitric oxide, thereby promoting endothelial dysfunction.
- MPO catalyzes the oxidation of HDL-C impairing its ability to perform reverse cholesterol transport.
- MPO catalyzes the oxidation of LDL-C contributing to foam cell formation and plaque progression.
- Elevated MPO levels predict risk for developing CAD in healthy individuals independent of traditional CVD risk factors.
- Elevated MPO levels contribute to plaque instability and are associated with increased risk of CVD events.

Relative Risk

20 X increased risk of CAD
5 X increased risk of MI (when negative for Troponin T)
2 X increase in all cause mortality

Causative Factors

Conditions
- History of chest pain
- Familial History of CHD
- Hypertension
- Myocardial infarction
- Peripheral arterial disease
- Stroke
- Atrial fibrillation

Therapeutic Options

Lifestyle
- Exercise
- Weight loss (as appropriate)
- Low fat diet

Medications
- Statin
- Aspirin
- Combination therapy
- Pioglitazone (if not contraindicated)
- Omega-3 fatty acid supplementation for anti-inflammatory and anti-oxidant effects
- Clopidogrel (Plavix®) if remote history of disease (particularly stent), prescription would be dependent on CYP2C19 genotype

Therapeutic Goal

< 400 pmol/L

Omega-3/Omega-6 Fatty Acid Profile Low HS-Omega-3 Index®

Disorder

- High risk range < 4%
- Intermediate risk range 4%—8%
- Optimal omega-3 fatty acid levels positively impact heart rate, blood pressure, triglyceride levels, myocardial efficiency, inflammatory responses, and endothelial function

Relative Risk

10 x increased risk for sudden cardiac death for < 4% vs. >8%

Causative Factors

- Low intake of omega-3 rich foods, particularly EPA+DHA (seafoods, mainly oily fish)

Therapeutic Options

- Increase intake of EPA+DHA from oily fish and/or fish oil supplements:
  - If HS-Omega-3 Index® 4%–8%: 0.5–1 g/day
  - If HS-Omega-3 Index® <4%: 1–2 g/day
- Retest in 4–6 months after titrating omega-3 dose

Therapeutic Goal

HS-Omega-3 Index® > 8%

Elevated Non-cholesterol Sterols

Disorder

- Sterols are crucial components of cell membranes in animals (zoosterols, namely cholesterol) and plants (phytosterols). Stanols are Δ5 saturated sterols
- Phytosterols serve no physiologic purpose in humans, are not readily absorbed, and cannot be synthesized
- They are present in small quantities in many fruits, vegetables, vegetable oils, nuts, seeds, cereals, and legumes

- Sitosterol, campesterol, and cholestanol (a stanol) are markers of cholesterol absorption; desmosterol is a marker of cholesterol synthesis
- Individual variation in cholesterol synthesis/absorption can help predict risk and affect the efficacy of lipid management therapy
- Elevations of plasma phytosterols may lead to atherogenesis and are powerful markers of CHD risk
- Elevated levels can identify patients with heterozygous or homozygous phytosterolemia or CTX

Optimal Range

Absorption mkrs:
  Values outside this range indicate hypo- (if <) or hyper- (if >) absorber
Campesterol
  2.11–4.43 μg/mL
Campesterol Ratio*
  114.55–239.77
Sitosterol
  1.43–3.17 μg/mL
Sitosterol Ratio*
  75.83–167.85
Cholestanol
  2.02–3.47 μg/mL
Cholestanol Ratio*
  116.87–194.27
Synthesis mkr:
  Values outside this range indicate hypo- (if <) or hyper- (if >) synthesizer
Desmosterol:
  0.50–1.27 μg/mL
Desmosterol Ratio*:
  31.02–64.43
  * ratios measured as 102 mmol sterol/stanol per mol cholesterol
  NB. Unless campesterol or sitosterol are in the ranges seen with phytosterolemic patients (100–300 μg/mL), one cannot state with assurance that the phytosterols are the cause of atherosclerotic plaque or events.

Causative Factors

Hypersynthetic or hyperabsorptive states:
- Common genetic variants affecting expression of NPC1L1 or causing defective ABCG5/ ABCG8 or heterozygous loss-of-function mutations

Hyperabsorptive states:
- Homozygous loss-of-function mutations in ABCG5/ABCG8 (phytos-terolemia)
- Over-expression of NPC1L1
- Post-menopause
- Family hx of premature CHD
- Type-2 diabetes or metabolic syndrome
- Statin (higher dose) monotherapy

Therapeutic Options

Medications:

To lower LDL-C/LDL-P levels in at-risk patients:
- Cholesterol synthesis can be reduced with a statin drug
- Cholesterol absorption can be reduced with ezetimibe, fenofibrate, or phytostanols
- Combination therapy (statins + ezetimibe) has the greatest LDL-lowering effects
- Ezetimibe (blocks absorption of all sterols) is also used to treat phytos-terolemia—combining with fenofibrate is more effective
- Esterifed sterols and stanols as dietary supplements—alone or with either a statin, ezetimibe, or bile acid sequestrant can enhance LDL lowering
- If phytosterol levels are elevated, only use a stanol (Benecol) instead of a phytosterol as a supplement

Therapeutic Goal

- Optimal cholesterol-lowering regimen personalized for each patient based on indicators of cholesterol metabolism
- Monitor absorption markers in patients on high dose statin monotherapy
- Monitor synthesis markers in patients on ezetimibe
- Monitor phytosterols in patients using sterol-containing nutritional supplements

Disclaimer

The HDL, Inc. Clinical Treatment Suggestions provide principles of practice that should produce high quality patient care and extend the continuum of care. It is intended for trained healthcare providers. The HDL, Inc. Clinical Treatment Suggestions should NOT be considered exclusive of other methods of care reasonably directed at obtaining positive results. The ultimate judgment concerning the propriety of any course of conduct must always be made by the clinician after careful consideration of each patient's individual situation.

Courtesy of Health Diagnostic Laboratory, Inc.

©2011 Health Diagnostic Laboratory, Inc.
1.877.4HDLABS (1.877.443.5227)
www.myhdl.com
737 N. 5th Street, Suite 103, Richmond, VA 23219
HDL-60.6 2011

Overview of Lipid Altering Medications

Drug Class	Specific Drug & Daily Dose	LDL-C	small dense LDL	HDL-C	HDL2	Triglycerides
Statins	Atorvastatin (Lipitor®) 10–80 mg	39–60% decrease	38–44% decrease	5–9% increase	24% increase	12–19% decrease
	Fluvastatin (Lescol®) 20–80 mg ALL PATIENTS	22–36% decrease	*	3–7% increase	+	17–25% decrease
	Fluvastatin (Lescol®) 20–80 mg PATIENTS w/TRIGLYCERIDES ≥ 200mg/dL	22–35% decrease	*	6–11% increase	+	12–25% decrease
	Lovastatin (Mevacor®) 20–40 mg	21–32% decrease	*	2–8% increase	+	6–10% decrease
	Pitavastatin (Livalo®) 1–4 mg	31–45% decrease	*	1–8% increase	*	13–20% decrease
	Pravastatin (Pravachol®) 10–80 mg	4–37% decrease	*	1–12% increase	+	4–24% decrease
	Rosuvastatin (Crestor®) 5–40 mg ALL PATIENTS	45–63% decrease	30% decrease	8–14% increase	+	10–35% decrease
	Rosuvastatin (Crestor®) 5–40 mg PATIENTS w/TRIGLYCERIDES ≥ 200mg/dL	26–47% decrease	30% decrease	3–22% increase	+	21–43% decrease
	Simvastatin (Zocor®) 5–80 mg	38–47% decrease	25% decrease	8–16% increase	42% increase	12–33% decrease
Niacin	(ER) Niacin (Niaspan®) 1–2 gm	9–17% decrease	43% decrease	15–26% increase	37% increase	16–38% decrease
	Crystalline (IR) niacin 1–6 gm	5–25% decrease	44% decrease	45% increase	36% increase	30% decrease
	Slow–release (SR) niacin 1–2 gm	5–25% decrease	*	5–15% increase	5% decrease	*

Class	Drug					
Fibrates	Fenofibrate (TriCor®) 145–200 mg	5–20% decrease	*	10–14% increase	+	20–50% decrease
	Fenofibric Acid (Trilipix®) 45–135 mg	5% decrease	*	16% increase	*	31% decrease
Fish Oil	Prescription fish oil (Lovaza®) 4 gm	49% increase	*	9% increase	+ dependent on ApoE Genotype.	50% decrease
	Non-Prescription fish oils 1–4 gm	no change or increase if high TRIG present	*	6–9% increase	+ dependent on ApoE Genotype.	45% decrease
Cholesterol Absorption Inhibitor	Ezetimibe (Zetia®) 10–80 mg	13–19% decrease	*	4% increase	*	11% decrease
Resins	Cholestyramine (Questran®) 4–16 gm	15–30% decrease	*	no effect	no effect	no change/increase
	Colestipol (Colestid®) 5–20 gm	15–30% decrease	*	no effect	no effect	no change/increase
	Colesevelam (WelChol®) 2.6–3.8 gm	15–18% decrease	*	3% increase	no effect	9% increase
Combination Drugs	Lovastatin/ERN (Advicor®) Available in 500/20mg, 750/20mg, 1000/20mg, 1000/40mg	30–42% decrease	*	20–30% increase	189% increase	30–40% decrease
	Simvastatin/ERN (SimCor®) Available in 500/20mg, 750/20mg, 1000/20mg	5–14% decrease	*	20–29% increase	+	22–38% decrease
	Ezetimibe/Simvastatin (Vytorin®) Available in 10/10mg, 10/20mg, 10/40mg, 10/80mg	45–60% decrease	*	8–10% increase	*	23–31% decrease

Bibliography
and Additional Reading

Week 1

American Dental Association, *www.ada.org*.

Become an Ex-Smoker, *www.becomeanex.org*.

Boffetta, P. and K. Straif, "Use of smokeless tobacco and risk of myocardial infarction and stroke: Systemic review with meta-analysis." *British Medical Journal*, Aug. 2009; 339: b3060.

Bullen, C. "Impact of tobacco smoking and smoking cessation on cardiovascular risk and disease." *Expert Review of Cardiovascular Therapy*, July 2008; 6(6): 883–895.

Erhardt L. "Cigarette smoking: An undertreated risk factor for cardiovascular disease." *Atherosclerosis*, July 2009; 205(1): 23–32.

Gerber, Y., L.J. Rosen, U. Goldbourt, Y. Benyamini, Y. Drory, et al. "Smoking status and long-term survival after first acute myocardial infarction: A population-based cohort study." *Journal of the American College of Cardiology*, Dec. 2009; 54(25): 2382–2387.

Glick, M. and B.L. Greenburg, "The potential role of dentists in indentifying patients' risk of experiencing coronary artery disease events." *Journal of the American Dental Association*, Nov. 2005; 136: 1541–1546.

Smokefree.gov, *http://smokefree.gov*.

Jontell, M. and M. Glick. "Oral health care professionals' identification of cardiovascular disease risk among patients in private dental offices in Sweden." *Journal of the American Dental Association*, Nov. 2009; 140(11): 1385–1391.

Piano, M.R., N.L. Benowitz, G.A. FitzGerald, et al. "Impact of smokeless tobacco products on cardiovascular disease." *Circulation*, Oct. 2010; 122(15):1520–44.

Strauss, S. et al. "The dental office visit as a potential opportunity for diabetes screening: An analysis using NHANES 2003–2004 data." *Journal of Public Health Dentistry*, Spring 2010; 70(2): 156–162.

Week 2

American College of Sports Medicine, *www.acsm.org*.

American Heart Association, *www.aha.org*.

252

Bassett, D. R., P.L. Schneider, and G.E. Huntington. "Physical activity in an Old Order Amish community." *Medical Science Sports Exercize*, Jan. 2004; 36(1): 79°85.

Chang, A.Y. et al. "Cardiovascular risk factors and coronary atherosclerosis in retired National Football League players." *American Journal of Cardiology* 2009; 104(6): 805–811.

Exercise is Medicine, *www.exerciseismedicine.org*.

Flynn, K.E. et al. "Effects of exercise training on health status in patients with chronic heart failure: HF-ACTION randomized controlled trial." *Journal of the American Medical Association*, 2009; 301(14): 1451–1459.

Hamburg, N.M., C.J. McMackin, et al. "Physical inactivity rapidly induces insulin resistance and microvascular dysfunction in healthy volunteers." *Arteriosclerosis, Thrombosis, & Vascular Biology*, Dec. 2007; 27(12): 2650–2656.

Hewitt, J.A., G.P. Whyte, et al. "The effects of a graduated aerobic exercise programme on cardiovascular disease risk factors in the NHS workplace: A randomised controlled trial." *Journal of Occupational Medical Toxicology*, Feb. 2008; 3:7.

Hunter, G.R. et al. "Exercise training prevents regain of visceral fat for 1 year following weight loss." *Obesity*, April 2010; 18(4): 690–695.

Kelley, G.A., K.A. Med Kelley, and Z.V. Tran. "Aerobic exercise and resting blood pressure: A meta-analytic review of randomized, controlled trials." *Preventive Cardiology* Spring 2001; 4(2): 73–80.

Keteyian, S. et al. American College of Cardiology's 58th Annual Scientific Session. Mar. 2009. Orlando, Florida.

———. "Exercise training in patients with heart failure." *Annals of Internal Medicine*, June 1996; 124(12): 1051–1057.

Kruger J., H.M. Blanck, and C. Gillespie. "Dietary and physical activity behaviors among adults successful at weight loss maintenance." *International Journal of Behavioral Nutrition and Physical Activity*, July 2006; 3:17.

Lalande, S. et al. "Effects of interval walking on physical fitness in middle-aged individuals." *Journal of Primary Care & Community*, July 2010; 1(2): 104–110.

Libby, P., R.O. Bonow, D.L. Mann, and D.P. Zipes. *Braunwald's Heart Disease: A Textbook of Cardiovascular Medicine*. Philadelphia: Saunders, 2007.

Madden, K.M., C. Lockhart, D. Cuff, et al. "Short-term aerobic exercise reduces arterial stiffness in older adults with Type 2 diabetes, hypertension and hypercholesterolemia." *Diabetes Care*, Aug. 2009; 32(8): 1531–1535.

Marieb, E. and K. Hoehn. *Human Anatomy & Physiology* (7th ed.). Pearson Benjamin Cummings (2007), 317.

Morris, J. "Vigorous exercise in leisure-time: Protection against coronary artery disease." *Journal of Epidemiology and Community Health*. Dec. 1978; 32(4): 239–243.

O'Connor, C.M. et al. "Efficacy and safety of exercise training in patients with chronic heart failure." *Journal of the American Medical Association*, 2009; 301(14): 1439–1450.

Paffenbarger, R.S., S.N. Blair, and I. Lee. "A history of physical activity, cardiovascular health and longevity: The scientific contributions of Jeremy N. Morris." *International Journal of Epidemiology* 2001; 30(5): 1184–1192.

Puetz, T.W., S.S. Flowers, and P.J. O'Connor. "A Randomized Controlled Trial of the Effect of Aerobic Exercise Training on Feelings of Energy and Fatigue in Sedentary Young Adults with Persistent Fatigue." *Psychotherapy and Psychosomatics*, Feb. 2008; 77(3): 167–174.

Rendi, M., A. Szabo, et al. "Acute psychological benefits of aerobic exercise: A field study into the effects of exercise characteristics." *Psychology, Health, and Medicine*, Mar. 2008; 13(2): 180–184.

Roussel, M. et al. "Influence of a walking program on the metabolic risk profile of obese postmenopausal women." *Menopause*, May/June 2009; 16(3): 566–575.

Sattelmair, J.R., T. Kurth, J.E. Buring, and I.M. Lee. "Physical activity and risk of stroke in women." *Stroke*, April 2010; 41(6): 1243.

Schjerve, I.E., G.A. Tyldum, et al. "Both aerobic endurance and strength training programs improve cardiovascular health in obese adults." *Clinical Science (London)*, Mar. 2008, 13.

Tudor-Locke, C. "Steps to better cardiovascular health: How many steps does it take to achieve good health and how confident are we in this number?" *Current Cardiovascular Risk Report*, 2010; 4: 271–276.

Week 3

American Association for Therapeutic Humor, *www.aath.org*.

Arthur, H.M., C. Patterson, and J.A. Stone. "The role of complementary and alternative therapies in cardiac rehabilitation: A systematic evaluation." *European Journal of Cardiovascular Preventative Rehabilitation* Feb. 2006; 13(1): 3–9.

Bennett, M.P. and C. Lengacher. "Humor and Laughter May Influence Health: III. Laughter and Health Outcomes." *Evidence-Based Complementary and Alternative Medicine*, Mar. 2008; 5(1): 37–40.

Das, S. and J.H. O'Keefe. "Behavioral cardiology: Recognizing and addressing the profound impact of psychosocial stress on cardiovascular health." *Current Atherosclerosis Report*, Mar. 2006; 8(2): 111–118.

Denollet, J., A. Schiffer, V. and Spek. "A general propensity to psychological distress affects cardiovascular outcomes: Evidence from research on Type D (distressed) personality profile." *Circulation: Cardiovascular Quality and Outcomes*, 2010; 3: 546–557.

Donga, E. et al. "A single night of partial sleep deprivation induces insulin resistance in multiple metabolic pathways in healthy subjects." *Journal of Clinical Endocrinology & Metabolism*, 2010; 95(6): 2963–2968.

Friedberg, J.P., S. Suchday, and D.V. Shelov. "The impact of forgiveness on cardiovascular reactivity and recovery." *International Journal of Psychophysiology*, Aug. 2007; 65(2): 87–94.

Karelina, K., et al. "Social isolation alters neuroinflammatory response to stroke." *Proceedings of the National Academy of Science*, April 2009; 106(14): 5895–5900.

Katzer, L., A.J. Bradshaw, et al. "Evaluation of a 'nondieting' stress reduction program for overweight women: A randomized trial." *American Journal of Health Promotion*, May–April 2008; 22(4): 264–274.

Kiecolt-Glaser, J.K. et al. "Stress, inflammation and yoga practice." *Psychosomatic Medicine*, 2010; 72: 1–9.

Kuntsevich, V., W.C. Bushell, and N.D. Theise. "Mechanisms of Yogic practices in health, aging and disease." *Mount Sinai Journal of Medicine*, Sept./Oct. 2010; 77(5): 559–569.

Kupper, N., Y. Gidron, J. Winter, and J. Denollet. "Association between Type D personality, depression, and oxidative stress in patients with chronic heart failure." *Psychosomatic Medicine*, 2009; 71: 973–980.

Laughter Yoga, *www.laughteryoga.org*.

Martens, E.J., F. Mols, M.M. Burg, and J. Denollet. "Type D personality and disease severity independently predict clinical events after myocardial infarction." *Journal of Clinical Psychiatry*, 2010; 71(6): 778–783.

Martens, E.J., P. de Jonge, B. Na, B.E. Cohen, H. Lett, and M.A. Whooley. "Scared to death? Generalized anxiety disorder and cardiovascular events in patients with stable coronary heart disease." *Archives of General Psychiatry*, 2010; 67(7): 750–758.

Matthews, K.A., B.B. Gump, et al. "Hostile behaviors predict cardiovascular mortality among men enrolled in the Multiple Risk Factor Intervention Trial." *Circulation*, Jan. 2004; 109(1): 66–70.

Miller, M. and W. Fry. "The effect of mirthful laughter on the human cardiovascular system." *Medical Hypotheses*, 2009; 73: 636–639.

Nabi, H. et al. "Effects of depressive symptoms and coronary heart disease and their interactive associations on mortality in middle-aged adults: The Whitehall II cohort study." *Heart*, Sept. 2010; doi:10.1136/hrt.2010.198507.

Naska, A., E. Oikonomou, A. Trichopoulou, T. Psaltopoulou, and D. Trichopoulos. "Siesta in healthy adults and coronary mortality in the general population." *Archives of Internal Medicine*, Feb. 2007; 167(3): 296–301.

Penson, R.T. and R.A. Partridge. "Laughter: The best medicine?" *Oncologist*, Sep. 2005; 10(8): 651–660.

Pullen, P.R. et al. "Benefits of yoga for African American heart failure patients." *Medicine & Science in Sports & Exercise*, April 2010; 42(4): 651–657.

Rafalson, L. et al. "Short sleep duration is associated with the development of impaired fasting glucose: The Western New York Health Study." *Annals of Epidemiology*, Dec. 2010; 20(12): 883–889.

Rainforth, M.V., R.H. Schneider, et al. "Stress Reduction Programs in Patients with Elevated Blood Pressure: A Systematic Review and Meta-analysis." *Current Hypertension Report*, Dec. 2007; 9(6): 520–528.

Ruberman, W., A.B. Weinblatt, J.D. Goldberg, and B.S. Chaudhary. "Psychosocial influences on mortality after myocardial infarction." *New England Journal of Medicine*, Aug. 1984; 311: 552–559.

Sabanayagam C; Shankar A. Sleep duration and cardiovascular disease: results from the National Health Interview Survey. *SLEEP* 2010;33(8):1037–1042.

Schneider, R.H., C.N. Alexander, et al. "Long-term effects of stress reduction on mortality in persons > or = 55 years of age with systemic hypertension." *American Journal of Cardiology*, May 2005; 95(9): 1060–1064.

Schneider, R., S. Nidich, J.M. Kotchen, T. Kotchen, C. Grim, M. Rainforth, C.G. King, and J. Salerno. "Effects of stress reduction on clinical events in African Americans with coronary heart disease: A randomized controlled trial." *Circulation*, 2009; 120: S461.

Sivasankaran, S., S. Pollard-Quintner, et al. "The effect of a six-week program of yoga and meditation on brachial artery reactivity: Do psychosocial interventions affect vascular tone?" *Clinical Cardiology*, Sept. 2006; 29(9): 393–398.

Stewart, J.C., K.L. Rand, M.F. Muldoon, and T.W. Kamarck. "A prospective evaluation of the directionality of the depression-inflammation relationship." *Brain, Behavior and Immunity*, Oct. 2009; 23(7): 936–944.

Streeter, C.C. et al. "Effects of Yoga Versus Walking on Mood, Anxiety, and Brain GABA Levels: A randomized controlled MRS study." *The Journal of Alternative and Complementary Medicine*, 2010; 16 (11): 1145 DOI: 10.1089/acm.2010.0007.

Sugawara, J., T. Tarumi, and H. Tanaka. "Effect of mirthful laughter on vascular function." *The American Journal of Cardiology*, Sept. 2010; 106(6): 856–859.

Uebelacker, L.A. et al. "Hatha yoga for depression: Critical review of the evidence for efficacy, plausible mechanisms of action, and directions for future research." *Journal of Psychiatric Practice*, Jan. 2010; 16(1): 22–33.

Vlachopoulos, C. et al. "Divergent effects of laughter and mental stress on arterial stiffness and central hemodynamics." *Psychosomatic Medicine*, Mar. 2009; doi:10.1097/PSY.0b013e318198dcd4.

Walters, K., G. Rait, I. Petersen, R. Williams, and I. Nazareth. "Panic disorder and risk of new onset coronary heart disease, acute myocardial infarction, and cardiac mortality: Cohort study using the general practice research database." *European Heart Journal*, Oct. 2008; 29(24); 2981–2988. doi:10.1093/eurheartj/ehn477.

Week 4

Allen, J.P., M. Nelson, and A. Alling. "The legacy of Biosphere 2 for the study of biospherics and closed ecological systems." *Advances in Space Research*, 2003 ;31(7): 1629–1639.

Arab, L., W. Liu, and D. Elashoff. "Both black and green tea consumption associated with reduced risk of stroke." *The FASEB Journal*, April 2009; 23 Meeting Abstract Supplement: 345.5.

Aronne, L.J. and K.K. Isoldi. "Overweight and obesity: Key components of cardiometabolic risk." *Clinical Cornerstone*, 2007; 8(3): 29–37.

Balk, E..M, A.H. Lichtenstein, et al. "Effects of omega-3 fatty acids on serum markers of cardiovascular disease risk: A systematic review." *Atherosclerosis*, Nov. 2006; 189(1): 19–30.

Berger, J.S., D.L. Brown, and R.C. Becker. "Low-dose aspirin in patients with stable cardiovascular disease: A meta-analysis." *American Journal of Medicine*, Jan. 2008; 121(1): 43–49.

Bernstein, A.M., Q. Sun, F.B. Hu, M.J. Stampfer, J.E. Manson, and W.C. Willett. "Major dietary protein sources and risk of coronary heart disease in women." *Circulation*, 2010; 122: 876–883.

Bibbins-Domingo, K. and P. Coxson. "Adolescent overweight and future adult coronary heart disease." *New England Journal of Medicine*, Dec. 2007; 357(23): 2371–2379.

Bray, G.A., S.J. Nielsen, and B.M. Popkin. "Consumption of high-fructose corn syrup in beverages may play a role in the epidemic of obesity." *American Journal of Clinical Nutrition*, April 2004; 79(4): 537–543.

Burke, B.E., R. Neuenschwander, and R.D. Olson. "Randomized, double-blind, placebo-controlled trial of coenzyme Q10 in isolated systolic hypertension." *South Medical Journal*, Nov. 2001; 94(11): 1112–1117.

City of Boston Public Health Commission statement of banning trans fats: *www.bphc. org/programs/cib/chronicdisease/heal/transfat/Pages/Home.aspx.* Accessed 1/21/11.

Colomer, R., R. Lupu, et al. "Giacomo Castelvetro's salads. Anti-HER2 oncogene nutraceuticals since the 17th century?" *Clinical and Translational Oncology* Jan. 2008; 10(1): 30–34.

Crawford, P. "Effectiveness of cinnamon for lowering hemoglobin A1C in patients with Type 2 diabetes: A randomized, controlled trial." *The Journal of the American Board of Family Medicine*, 2009; 22(5): 507–512.

Crowe, F.L., A.W. Roddam, T.J. Key, et al. "Fruit and vegetable intake and mortality from ischaemic heart disease: Results from the European Prospective Investigation into Cancer and Nutrition (EPIC)-Heart study." *European Heart Journal*, Jan. 2011; 32. doi: 10.1093/eurheartj/ehq465.

Dai, J., R. Lampert, P.W. Wilson, J. Goldberg, T.R. Ziegler, and V. Vaccarino. "Mediterranean dietary pattern is associated with improved cardiac autonomic function among middle-aged men." *Circulation: Cardiovascular Quality and Outcomes*, June 2010.

Daniel, C.R., A.J. Cross, C. Koebnick, and R. Sinha. "Trends in red meat consumption in the USA." *Public Health Nutrition*, published online Nov. 2010.

Dannenberg, A.L., D.C. Burton, R.J. Jackson. "Economic and environmental costs of obesity: The impact on airlines." *American journal of preventive medicine* 2004; 27 (3): 264. doi:10.1016/j.amepre.2004.06.004

Degirolamo, C., G.S. Shelness, and L.L. Rudel. "LDL cholesteryl oleate as a predictor for atherosclerosis: Evidence from human and animal studies on dietary fat." *The Journal of Lipid Research*, April 2009; 50: S434–S439.

Djoussé, L. and J.M. Gaziano. "Alcohol consumption and risk of heart failure in the Physicians' Health Study I." *Circulation*, Jan. 2007; 115(1) :34–39.

Djousse, L., P.N. Hopkins, K.E. North, J.S. Pankow, D.K. Arnett, and R.C. Ellison. "Chocolate consumption is inversely associated with prevalent coronary heart disease: The National Heart, Lung, and Blood Institute Family Heart Study." *Clinical Nutrition*. Article in press at time of publishing.

Egan, J.M. and R.F. Margolskee. "Taste cells of the gut and gastrointestinal chemosensation." *Molecular Interventions*, April 2008; 8(2): 78–81.

Ellis, E.M. "Reactive carbonyls and oxidative stress: Potential for therapeutic intervention." *Pharmacology & Therapeutics*, July 2007; 115(1): 13–24.

Ello-Martin, J.A., J.H. Ledikwe, and B.J. Rolls. "The influence of food portion size and energy density on energy intake: Implications for weight management." *American Journal of Clinical Nutrition*, July 2005; 82(1 Suppl): 236S–241S.

Engler, M.M. and M.B. Engler. "Omega-3 fatty acids: Role in cardiovascular health and disease." *Journal of Cardiovascular Nursing*, Jan–Feb 2006; 21(1): 17–24, quiz 25–26.

Folts, J.D. "The history of aspirin." *Texas Heart Institute Journal*, 2007; 34(3): 392.

Fontana, L. "Calorie restriction and cardiometabolic health." *European Journal of Cardiovascular Preventative Rehabilitation*, Feb. 2008; 15(1): 3–9.

Fontana, L. "Nutrition, adiposity and health." *Epidemiology Prevention*, Sep.–Oct. 2007; 31(5): 290–294.

Forshee, R.A., M..L. Storey, et al. "A critical examination of the evidence relating high fructose corn syrup and weight gain." *Critical Reviews in Food Science & Nutrition*, 2007; 47(6): 561–582.

Freiberg, M.S., M.J. Pencina, R.B. D'Agostino, K. Lanier, P.W. Wilson, and R.S. Vasan. "BMI vs. waist circumference for identifying vascular risk." *Obesity*, 2008; 16: 463–469.

Fung, T.T., K.M. Rexrode, C.S. Mantzoros, J.E. Manson, W.C. Willett, and F.B. Hu. "Mediterranean diet and incidence of and mortality from coronary heart disease and stroke in women." *Circulation*, 2009; 119: 1093–1100.

Gaby, A.R. "Adverse effects of dietary fructose." *Alternative Medicine Review*, Dec. 2005; 10(4): 294–306.

Harris, W.S. "Omega-3 fatty acids and cardiovascular disease: A case for omega-3 index as a new risk factor." *Pharmacological Research*, Mar. 2007; 55(3): 217–223.

Hayman, L.L., J.C. Meininger, et al. "Primary prevention of cardiovascular disease in nursing practice: Focus on children and youth." *Circulation*, 2007; 116: 344–357.

Holick, M.F. and T.C. Chen. "Vitamin D deficiency: A worldwide problem with health consequences." *American Journal of Clinical Nutrition*, April 2008; 87(4): 1080S–1806S.

Houston, M.C. "Treatment of hypertension with nutraceuticals, vitamins, antioxidants and minerals." *Expert Review of Cardiovascular Therapy*, July 2007; 5(4): 681–691.

Jacobs Jr., D.R., L.F. Andersen, and R. Blomhoff. "Whole-grain consumption is associated with a reduced risk of noncardiovascular, noncancer death attributed to inflammatory diseases in the Iowa Women's Health Study." *American Journal of Clinical Nutrition*, June 2007; 85(6): 1606–1614.

Jalal, D.I. and T. Ikizler. "High fructose consumption is independently associated with high blood pressure." Renal Week: American Society of Nephrology (ASN) 2009 Annual Meeting: Abstract TH-FC037.

Janson, M. "Orthomolecular medicine: The therapeutic use of dietary supplements for anti-aging." *Journal of Clinical Interventions in Aging*, 2006 ;1(3): 261–265.

Keys, A. "Mediterranean diet and public health: personal reflections." *merican Journal of Clinical Nutrition*, June 1995; 61(6 Suppl): 1321S–1323S.

Knoops, K.T., L.C. de Groot, et al. "Mediterranean diet, lifestyle factors, and 10-year mortality in elderly European men and women: The HALE project." *Journal of the American Medical Association*, Sep. 2004; 292(12): 1433–1439.

Konstantinidou, V., M.I. Covas, et al. "In vivo nutrigenomic effects of virgin olive oil polyphenols within the frame of the Mediterranean diet: A randomized controlled trial." *The FASEB Journal*, July 2010; 24(7): 2546–2557.

Konukoğlu, D. and G.D. Kemerli. "Protein carbonyl content in erythrocyte membranes in type 2 diabetic patients." *Hormone & Metabolic Research*, July 2002; 34(7): 367–370.

Lam, T.K., A.J. Cross, D. Consonni, G. Randi, V. Bagnardi, P.B. Bertazzi, N.E. Caporaso, R. Sinha, A.F. Subar, and M.T. Landi. "Intakes of red meat, processed meat and meat mutagens increase lung cancer risk." *Cancer Research*, 2009; 69: 932.

Lin, B.H., J. Guthrie, and E. Frazao. "Nutrient contribution of food away from home." In: Frazao, E. (Ed.), *America's Eating Habits: Changes and Consequences*. Agriculture Information Bulletin No. 750, 1999: US Department of Agriculture, Economic Research Service, Washington, D.C., 213–239.

Malik, V.S., M.B. Schulze, and F.B. Hu. "Intake of sugar-sweetened beverages and weight gain: A systematic review." *American Journal of Clinical Nutrition*, Aug. 2006; 84(2): 274–288.

Mancini, M., and J. Stamler. "Diet for preventing cardiovascular diseases: Light from Ancel Keys, distinguished centenarian scientist." *Nutrition, Metabolism & Cardiovascular Disease*, Feb. 2004; 14(1): 52–57.

Martini, L.A. and R.J Wood. "Vitamin D and blood pressure connection: Update on epidemiologic, clinical, and mechanistic evidence." *Nutritional Review*, May 2008; 66(5): 291–297.

Maser, R.E. and M.J. Lenhard. "An overview of the effect of weight loss on cardiovascular autonomic function." *Current Diabetes Review*, Aug. 2007; 3(3): 204–211.

Mayo Clinic Health Information. "Artificial Sweeteners: Understanding these and other sugar substitutes." *www.mayoclinic.com/health/artificial-sweeteners/MY00073*. Accessed 1/21/11.

Micha, R., S.K. Wallace, D. Mozaffarian. "Red and processed meat consumption and risk of incident coronary heart disease, stroke and diabetes mellitus." *Circulation*, 2010; 121: 2271–2283.

Miner, J. and A. Hoffhines. "The discovery of aspirin's antithrombotic effects." *Texas Heart Institute Journal*, 2007 ;34(2): 179–186.

Mitrou, P.N., V. Kipnis, et al. "Mediterranean dietary pattern and prediction of all-cause mortality in a US population: Results from the NIH-AARP Diet and Health Study." *Archives of Internal Medicine*, Dec. 2007; 167(22): 2461–2468.

Morrill, A.C. and C.D. Chinn. "The obesity epidemic in the United States." *Journal of Public Health Policy*, 2004; 25(3–4): 353–366.

Mozaffarian, D. "Trans fatty acids—effects on systemic inflammation and endothelial function." *Atherosclerosis Supplement*, May 2006; 7(2): 29–32.

Nakanishi, Y., K. Tsuneyama, et al. "Monosodium glutamate (MSG): A villain and pro-moter of liver inflammation and dysplasia." *Journal of Autoimmunology*, Feb.–Mar. 2008; 30(1–2): 42–50.

New York City Department of Health and Mental Hygiene, Statement on Trans Fats: *www.nyc.gov/html/doh/html/cardio/cardio-transfat.shtml*. Accessed 1/21/11.

Nilsson, M., J. Holst, and I. Bjorck. "Metabolic effects of amino acid mixtures and whey protein in healthy subjects: Studies using glucose-equivalent drinks." *American Journal of Clinical Nutrition*, 2007; 85: 996–1004.

Odetti, P., S. Garibaldi, et al. "Levels of carbonyl groups in plasma proteins of type 2 diabetes mellitus subjects." *Acta Diabetologica*. Dec. 1999; 36(4): 179–183.

O'Keefe, J.H., N.M. Gheewala, and J.O. O'Keefe. "Dietary strategies for improving post-prandial glucose, lipids, inflammation, and cardiovascular health." *Journal of the American College of Cardiology*, Jan. 2008; 51(3): 249–255.

O'Keefe, T., K. Bybee, and C. Lavie. "Alcohol and cardiovascular health: The razor-sharp double-edge sword." *Journal of the American College of Cardiology*, 2007; 50(11): 1009–1014.

Ostman, E., Y. Granfeldt, L. Persson, and I. Bjorck. "Vinegar supplementation lowers glucose and insulin responses and increases satiety after a bread meal in healthy subjects." *European Journal of Clinical Nutrition*, 2005; 59: 983–988.

Ozner, M. *The Miami Mediterranean Diet* 2nd Edition. Dallas, TX: BenBella Books, 2008.

Pennathur, S. and J.W. Heinecke. "Mechanisms for oxidative stress in diabetic cardio-vascular disease." *Antioxidants & Redox Signaling*, July 2007; 9(7): 955–969.

Pennathur, S., Y. Ido, et al. "Reactive carbonyls and polyunsaturated fatty acids pro-duce a hydroxyl radical-like species: A potential pathway for oxidative damage of retinal proteins in diabetes." *Journal of Biological Chemistry*, June 2005; 280(24): 22706–22714.

Pergams, O.R. and P.A. Zaradic. "Evidence for a fundamental and pervasive shift away from nature-based recreation." *Proceedings of the National Academy of Sciences of the United States of America*, Feb. 2008.

Pitsavos, C., D.B. Panagiotakos, et al. "Forty-year follow-up of coronary heart dis-ease mortality and its predictors: The Corfu cohort of the seven countries study." *Preventative Cardiology*, Summer 2003; 6(3): 155–160.

Pradhan, A. "Obesity, metabolic syndrome, and type 2 diabetes: Inflammatory ba-sis of glucose metabolic disorders." *Nutritional Review*, Dec. 2007; 65(12 Pt 2): S152–S156.

Puangsombat, K. and J.S. Smith. "Inhibition of heterocyclic amine formation in beef patties by ethanolic extracts of rosemary." *Journal of Food Science*, Mar. 2010; 75(2): T40–T47.

Reaven, G., F. Abbasi, and T. McLaughlin. "Obesity, insulin resistance, and cardiovas-cular disease." *Recent Progress in Hormone Resistance*, 2004; 59: 207–223.

Ried, K., T. Sullivan, P. Fakler, O.R. Frank, and N.P. Stocks. "Does chocolate reduce blood pressure? A meta-analysis." *BMC Medicine*, 2010; 8(39).

Rosito, G.A., J.M. Massaro, U. Hoffman, F.L. Ruberg, A.A. Mahabadi, C. J. O'Donnell, and C.S. Fox. "Pericardial fat, visceral abdominal fat, cardiovascular disease risk factors, and vascular calcification in a community-based sample." *Circulation*, 2008; 117: 605–613.

Sakata, Y., H. Zhuang, H. Kwansa, R.C. Koehler, and S. Dore. "Resveratrol protects against experimental stroke: Putative neuroprotective role of heme oxygenase 1." *Experimental Neurology*, July 2010; 224(1): 325–329.

Sanchez-Villegas, A., M. Delgado-Rodriguez, et al. "Association of the Mediterranean dietary pattern with the incidence of depression: The Seguimento Universidad de Navarra cohort." *Archives of General Psychiatry*, 2009; 66(10): 1090–1098.

Scarmeas, N., J.A. Luchsinger, N. Schupf, A.M. Brickman, S. Cosentino, M.X. Tang, and Y. Stern. "Physical activity, diet and risk of Alzheimer disease." *Journal of the American Medical Association*, 2009; 302(6): 627–637.

Scarmeas, N., Y. Stern, R. Mayeux, J.J. Manly, N. Schupf, and J.A. Luchsinger. "Mediterranean diet and mild cognitive impairment." *Archives of Neurology*, 2009; 66(2): 216–225.

Schwalfenberg, G. "Omega-3 fatty acids: Their beneficial role in cardiovascular health." *Canadian Family Physician*, June 2006; 52: 734–740.

Smith, J.S., F. Ameri, and P. Gadgil. "Effect of marinades on the formation of heterocyclic amines in grilled beef steaks." *Journal of Food Science*, April 2008; 73(6): T100–T105.

Soriano-Guillen, L., B. Hernandez-Garcia, et al. "High Sensitivity Creative Protein Is a Good Marker of Cardiovascular Risk Factor in Obese Children and Adolescents." *European Journal of Endocrinology*, May 2008.

State of California statement on banning of trans fats: *http://cchealth.org/groups/ eh/retail_food/pdf/ab97_transfat_ban_guidelines.pdf*. Accessed 1/21/11.

Steck, S.E. and J.R. Hebert. "GST polymorphism and excretion of heterocyclic aromatic amine and isothiocyanate metabolites after Brassica consumption." *Environmental and Molecular Mutagenesis*, April 2009; 50(3): 238–246.

Sun, Q., D. Spiegelman, R.M. van Dam, M.D. Holmes, V.S. Malik, W.C. Willett, and F.B. Hu. "White rice, brown rice and risk of Type 2 diabetes in US men and women." *Archives of Internal Medicine*. 2010; 170(11): 961–969.

Tapsell, L.C., I. Hemphill, et al. "Health benefits of herbs and spices: The past, the present, the future." *Medical Journal of Australia* Aug. 2006; 185(4 Suppl): S4–S24.

Teff, K.L., S.S. Elliott, et al. "Dietary fructose reduces circulating insulin and leptin, attenuates postprandial suppression of ghrelin, and increases triglycerides in women." *Journal of Clinical Endocrinology & Metabolism*, June 2004;89(6): 2963–2972.

Tiano, L., R. Belardinelli, et al. "Effect of coenzyme Q10 administration on endothelial function and extracellular superoxide dismutase in patients with ischaemic heart disease: A double-blind, randomized controlled study." *European Heart Journal*, Sep. 2007; 28(18): 2249–2255.

Trichopoulou, A. "Mediterranean diet: The past and the present." *Nutrition, Metabolism & Cardiovascular Disease*, Aug. 2001; 11(4 Suppl): 1–4.

Trichopoulou, A., C. Bamia, P. Lagiou, D. Trichopoulos. "Conformity to traditional Mediterranean diet and breast cancer risk in the Greek EPIC (European

Prospective Investigation into Cancer and Nutrition) cohort." *American Journal of Clinical Nutrition*, Sept. 2010; 92(3): 620–625.

Vieth, R., H. Bischoff-Ferrari, et al. "The urgent need to recommend an intake of vitamin D that is effective." *American Journal of Clinical Nutrition*, Mar. 2007; 85(3): 649–650.

Walford, R.L., D. Mock, et al. "Calorie restriction in biosphere 2: Alterations in physiologic, hematologic, hormonal, and biochemical parameters in humans restricted for a 2-year period." *Journals of Gerontology, Series A: Biological Science & Medical Science*, June 2002; 57(6): B211–224.

Wang, T.J., M.J. Pencina, et al. "Vitamin D deficiency and risk of cardiovascular disease." *Circulation*, Jan. 2008; 117(4): 503–511.

Wang, Z., B. Zhou, Y. Wang, Q. Gong, Q. Wang, J. Yan, W. Gao, and L. Wang. "Black and green tea consumption and the risk of coronary artery disease: A meta-analysis." *American Journal of Clinical Nutrition*, Mar. 2011; 93(3): 506–515.

Waterman, E. and B. Lockwood. "Active components and clinical applications of olive oil." *Alternative Medicine Review*, Dec. 2007; 12(4): 331–342.

Wu, X., J. Lin, et al. "Meat, especially if it's well done, may increase risk of bladder cancer." *ScienceDaily*, *www.sciencedaily.com/releases/2010/04/100419150827.htm*. Accessed January 22, 2011.

Yusuf, S., S. Hawken, S. Ounpuu, et al. "INTER-HEART study investigators. Effect of potentially modifiable risk factors associated with myocardial infarction in 52 countries (the INTER-HEART study): Case-control study." *Lancet*, 2004; 364: 937–952.

Week 5

Adhami, V.M., A. Malik, et al. "Combined Inhibitory Effects of Green Tea Polyphenols and Selective Cyclooxygenase-2 Inhibitors on the Growth of Human Prostate Cancer Cells Both In vitro and In vivo." *Clinical Cancer Research, Mar.* 2007; 13: 1611–1619.

Agusti, A. and J.B. Soriano. "COPD as a Systemic Disease." *COPD*, April 2008; 5(2): 133–138.

Ahmed, S., A. Pakozdi, et al. "Regulation of interleukin-1beta-induced chemokine production and matrix metalloproteinase 2 activation by epigallocatechin-3-gallate in rheumatoid arthritis synovial fibroblasts." *Arthritis & Rheumatism*, Aug. 2006; 54(8): 2393–2401.

Alyan, O., F. Kacmaz, et al. "Effects of Cigarette Smoking on Heart Rate Variability and Plasma N-Terminal Pro-B-Type Natriuretic Peptide in Healthy Subjects: Is There the Relationship between Both Markers?" *Annual Noninvasive Electrocardiology*, April 2008; 13(2): 137–144.

Araujo, J.A., B. Barajas, M. Kleinman, X. Wang, B.J. Bennett, K.W. Gong, M. Navab, J. Azadzoi, K.M., R.N. Schulman, et al. "Oxidative stress in arteriogenic erectile dysfunction: prophylactic role of antioxidants." *Journal of Urology*, July 2005; 174(1): 386–393.

Bauer, M., S. Moebus, S. Mohlenkamp, N. Dragano, M. Nonnemacher, M. Fuchsluger, C. Kessler, H. Jakobs, M. Memmesheimer, R. Erbel, K.H. Jockel, and B. Hoffman. "Urban particulate matter air pollution is associated with subclinical atherosclerosis: results from the HNR (Heinz Nixdorf Recall) study." *Journal of American College of Cardiology*, Nov. 2010; 56(23): 1803–1808.

Bear Jack Gebhardt. *The Enlightened Smoker's Guide to Quitting* 1ˢᵗ ed. Dallas, TX: BenBella Books, 2008.

Biswas, S. and I. Rahman. "Modulation of steroid activity in chronic inflammation: A novel anti-inflammatory role for curcumin." *Molecular Nutrition & Food Research*, Mar. 2008.

Bonomini, F.,S. Tengattini, et al. "Atherosclerosis and oxidative stress." *Histol Histopathol*, Mar. 2008; 23(3): 381–390.

Brown, M.K., J.L. Evans, et al. "Beneficial effects of natural antioxidants EGCG and alpha-lipoic acid on life span and age-dependent behavioral declines in Caenorhabditis elegans." *Pharmacology, Biochemistry and Behavior*, Nov. 2006; 85(3): 620–8.

Charrier-Hisamuddin, L., C.L. Laboisse, and D. Merlin. "ADAM-15: A metalloprotease that mediates inflammation." *The FASEB Journal*, Mar. 2008; 22(3): 641–53.

Chilton, F.H. and L.L. Rudel. :Mechanisms by which botanical lipids affect inflammatory disorders." *American Journal of Clinical Nutrition*, Feb. 2008; 87(2): 498S–503S.

Cipollone, F., A. Mezzetti, et al. "Association between 5-lipoxygenase expression and plaque instability in humans." *Arteriuscleriosis, Thrombosis & Vascular Biology*, Aug. 2005; 25(8): 1665–1670.

Cromwell, W.C. et al. "LDL Particle Number and Risk of Future Cardiovascular Disease in the Framingham Offspring Study—Implications for LDL Management." *Journal of Clinical Lipidology*, Dec. 2007; 1(6): 583–592.

Cuaz-Pérolin, C., L. Billiet, et al. "Anti-inflammatory and antiatherogenic effects of the NF-kappaB inhibitor acetyl-11-keto-beta-boswellic acid in LPS-challenged ApoE-/- mice." *Arteriosclerosis, Thrombosis and Vascular Biology*, Feb. 2008; 28(2): 272–277.

Davis, D.R. and J.H. Erlich. "Cardiac tissue factor: Roles in physiology and fibrosis." *Clinical and Experimental Pharmacology and Physiology*, Mar. 2008; 35(3): 342–348.

Engler, M.B., M.M. Engler, et al. "Flavonoid-rich dark chocolate improves endothelial function and increases plasma epicatechin concentrations in healthy adults." *Journal of the American College of Nutrition*, June 2004; 23(3): 197–204.

Erridge, C. "The roles of pathogen-associated molecular patterns in atherosclerosis." *Trends in Cardiovascular Medicine*, Feb. 2008; 18(2): 52–56.

Forest, C.P., H. Padma-Nathan, H.R. Liker. "Efficacy and safety of pomegranate juice on improvement of erectile dysfunction in male patients with mild to moderate erectile dysfunction: A randomized, placebo-controlled, double-blind, crossover study. *International Journal of Impotence Research*, Nov.–Dec. 2007; 19(6): 564–567.

Gawaz, M. "Platelets in the onset of atherosclerosis." *Blood Cells, Molecules & Diseases*, Mar.–April 2006; 36(2): 206–210.

Gerry, J.M. and G. Pascual. "Narrowing in on Cardiovascular Disease: The Atheroprotective Role of Peroxisome Proliferator-Activated Receptor gamma." *Trends in Cardiovascular Medicine*, Feb. 2008; 18(2): 39–44.

Ghamin, H., C>L. Sia, S. Abuaysheh, K. Korzeniewski, P. Patnaik, A. Marumganti, A. Chaudhuri, and P. Dandone. "An anti-inflammatory and reactive oxygen species suppressive effects of an extract of *Polygonum Cuspidatum* containing resveratrol." *Journal of Clinical Endocrinology & Metabolism*, 2010; 95(9): E1–E8.

Goel, A., A.B. Kunnumakkara, and B.B. Aggarwal. "Curcumin as 'Curecumin': From kitchen to clinic." *Biochemical Pharmacology*, Feb. 2008; 75(4): 787–809.

Gorelik, S., M. Ligumsky, R. Koehn, and J. Kanner. "A novel function of red wine polyphenols in humans: prevention of absorption of cytotoxic lipid peroxidation products." *The FASEB Journal*, Jan. 2008; 22(1): 41–46.

Harkema, C. Sioutas, A.J. Lusis and A.E., Nel. "Ambient particulate pollutants in the ultrafine range promote early atherosclerosis and system oxidative stress." *Circulation Research*, 2008; 102: 589–596.

Harman, D. "Free radical theory of aging. *Mutation Research*, Sept. 1992; 275(3–6): 257–266.

Harvard Medical School Publication on Glycemic Index: *www.health.harvard.edu/news-week/Glycemic_index_and_glycemic_load_for_100_foods.htm.* Accessed 1/21/11.

Hatcher, H., R. Planalp, et al. "Curcumin: From ancient medicine to current clinical trials." *Cellular & Molecular Life Sciences*, Mar. 2008.

Higuera-Ciapara, I., L. Felix-Valenzuela, et al. "Astaxanthin: A review of its chemistry and applications." *Critical Reviews in Food Science & Nutrition*, 2006; 46(2): 185–196.

Hussein G, Sankawa U, et al. Astaxanthin, a carotenoid with potential in human health and nutrition. *J Nat Prod.* 2006 Mar.;69(3):443-9.

Ide, R., Y. Fujino, et al. "A Prospective Study of Green Tea Consumption and Oral Cancer Incidence in Japan." *Annual Epidemiology*, June 2007.

Karlsson, K., B. Ahlborg, C. Dalman, and T. Hemmingsson. "Association between erythrocyte sedimentation rate and IQ in Swedish males aged 18–20." *Brain, Behavior and Immunity*, Aug. 2010; 24(6): 868–873.

Kaufman. "Long-term exposure to air pollution and incidence of cardiovascular events in women." *New England Journal of Medicine*, Feb. 2007; 356: 447–458.

Kuhn, H., P. Chaitidis, et al. "Arachidonic Acid metabolites in the cardiovascular system: The role of lipoxygenase isoforms in atherogenesis with particular emphasis on vascular remodeling." *Journal of Cardiovascular Pharmacology*, Dec. 2007; 50(6): 609–620.

Lancaster, T. and L. Stead. "Physician advice for smoking cessation." *Cochrane Database System Review*, Oct. 2004; (4): CD000165.

Li, L. and N.P. Seeram. "Maple syrup phytochemicals include lignans, coumaris, a stilbene, and other previously unreported antioxidant phenolic compounds." *Journal of Agriculture and Food Chemistry*, 2010; 58(22): 11673–11679.

Libby, P. "Inflammatory mechanisms: the molecular basis of inflammation and disease." *Nutritional Review*, Dec. 2007; 65(12 Pt 2): S140–S146.

Libby, P., P.M. Ridker, and A. Maseri. "Inflammation and atherosclerosis." *Circulation*, Mar. 2002; 105(9): 1135–1143.

Lovely, R.S., S.C. Kazmierczak, J.M. Massaro, R.B. D'Agostino, Sr., C.J. O'Donnell, and D.H. Farrell. "Gamma Fibrinogen: Evaluation of a New Assay for Study of Associations with Cardiovascular Disease." *Clinical Chemistry*, 2010; 56: 781–788.

Lucini, D., F. Bertocchi, et al. "A controlled study of the autonomic changes produced by habitual cigarette smoking in healthy subjects." *Cardiovascular Research*, April 1996; 31(4): 633–639.

May, A.E., P. Seizer, and M. Gawaz. "Platelets: inflammatory firebugs of vascular walls." *Arterioscleriosis, Thrombosis, & Vascular Biology*, Mar. 2008; 28(3): s5–10.

Miller, K.A., D.S. Siscovick, L. Sheppard, K. Shepherd, J.H. Sullivan, G.L. Anderson, and J.D. Villareal-Calderon, R., J. Palacios-Moreno, K. Parker, and L. Calderon-Garciduenas. "Gene inflammatory expression profiling in right versus left ventricles in young urbanites: What is the long-term impact of myocardial inflammation in the setting of air pollution?" *The FASEB Journal*, April 2010; 24 Meeting Abstract Supplement, 1029.1

Murphy, M.P. and R.A. Smith. "Targeting antioxidants to mitochondria by conjugation to lipophilic cations." *Annual Review of Pharmacological Toxicology*, 2007; 47: 629–656.

National Cholesterol Education Program:. *www.nhlbi.nih.gov/about/ncep*. Accessed 1/21/11.

Nissen, S.E., S.J. Nicholls, et al. "Effects of very high-intensity statin therapy on regression of coronary atherosclerosis." *Journal of the American Medical Association*, 2006; 295(13): 1556–1565.

O'Keefe, J.H., N.M. Gheewala, and J.O. O'Keefe. "Dietary strategies for improving postprandial glucose, lipids, inflammation, and cardiovascular health." *Journal of the America College of Cardiology*, Jan. 2008; 51(3): 249–255.

Packard, R.R. and P. Libby. "Inflammation in atherosclerosis: from vascular biology to biomarker discovery and risk prediction." *Clinical Chemistry*, Jan. 2008; 54(1): 24–38.

Papatheodorou, L. and N. Weiss. "Vascular oxidant stress and inflammation in hyperhomocysteinemia." *Antioxidants & Redox Signaling*, Nov. 2007; 9(11): 1941–1958.

Pearson, J.F., C. Bachireddy, S. Shyamprasad, A.B. Godlfine, and J.S. Brownstein. "Association between fine particulate matter and diabetes prevalence in the U.S." *Diabetes Care*, Oct. 2010; 33(10): 2196–2201.

Prior, R.L., L. Gu, et al. "Plasma antioxidant capacity changes following a meal as a measure of the ability of a food to alter in vivo antioxidant status." *Journal of the American College of Nutrition*, April 2007; 26(2): 170–181.

Ridker, P., E. Danielson, F. Fonseca, J. Genest, et al. "Reduction in C-reactive protein and LDL cholesterol and cardiovascular event rates after initiation of rosuvastatin: A prospective study of the JUPITER trial." *The Lancet*, 2009; 373(9670): 1175–1182.

Rizzo, M., E. Corrado, et al. "Prediction of cardio- and cerebro-vascular events in patients with subclinical carotid atherosclerosis and low HDL-cholesterol." *Atherosclerosis*, Feb. 2008.

Schleicher, E. and U. Friess. "Oxidative stress, AGE, and atherosclerosis." *Kidney International Supplement*, Aug. 2007; (106): S17–S26.

Seeram, N.P., M. Aviram, et al. "Comparison of Antioxidant Potency of Commonly Consumed Polyphenol-Rich Beverages in the United States." *Journal of Agricultural & Food Chemistry*, Feb. 2008; 56(4): 1415–1422.

Silverman, R.A., K. Ito, J. Freese, B.J. Kaufman, D. De Claro, J. Braun, and D.J. Prezant. "Association of ambient fine particles with out-of-hospital cardiac arrests in New York City." *American Journal of Epidemiology*, Aug. 2010. doi: 10.1093/aje/kwq217 *http://aje.oxfordjournals.org/content/early/2010/08/20/aje.kwq217.full. pdf+html*. Accessed 1/21/11.

Singh, S., A. Khajuria, et al. "Boswellic acids: A leukotriene inhibitor also effective through topical application in inflammatory disorders." *Phytomedicine*, Jan. 2008.

Smith, R.N., N.J. Mann, et al. "The effect of a high-protein, low glycemic-load diet versus a conventional, high glycemic-load diet on biochemical parameters associated with acne vulgaris: A randomized, investigator-masked, controlled trial. *Journal of the American Academy of Dermatology*, Aug. 2007; 57(2): 247–256.

Son, S.M.. "Role of vascular reactive oxygen species in development of vascular abnormalities in diabetes." *Diabetes Research and Clinical Practice*, Sept. 2007; 77 Supplement 1: S65–S70.

Tan, K.T. and G.Y. Lip. "Imaging of the unstable plaque." *International Journal of Cardiology*, Jan. 2008.

Taubert, D., R. Roesen, et al. "Effects of low habitual cocoa intake on blood pressure and bioactive nitric oxide: A randomized controlled trial." *Journal of the American Medical Association*, July 2007; 298(1): 49–60.

Thangapazham. R.L., A.K. Singh, et al. "Green tea polyphenols and its constituent epigallocatechin gallate inhibits proliferation of human breast cancer cells in vitro and in vivo." *Cancer Letters*, Jan. 2007; 245(1–2): 232–241.

Viera, L., K. Chen, A. Nel, and M.G. Lloret. "The impact of air pollutants as an adjuvant for allergic sensitization and asthma." *Current Allergy and Asthma Reports*, 2009; 9(4): 327–333.

Weinreb, O., S. Mandel, et al. "Neurological mechanisms of green tea polyphenols in Alzheimer's and Parkinson's diseases." *Journal of Nutritional Biochemistry*, Sept. 2004; 15(9): 506–516.

Wolfram, S., D. Raederstorff, et al. "Epigallocatechin gallate supplementation alleviates diabetes in rodents." *Journal of Nutrition*, Oct. 2006; 136(10): 2512–25128.

Yamagishi. S., T. Matsui, K. Nakamura. "Possible involvement of tobacco-derived advanced glycation end products (AGEs) in an increased risk for developing cancers and cardiovascular disease in former smokers." *Medical Hypotheses*, April 2008.

Yasuda, O. and Y. Takemura. "Aspirin: Recent developments." *Cellular Molecular Life Science*, Feb. 2008; 65(3): 354–358.

Yusuf, N., C. Irby, et al. "Photoprotective effects of green tea polyphenols." *Photodermatology, Photoimmunology, & Photomedicine*, Feb. 2007; 23(1): 48–56.

Week 6

Anderson, J.L., H.T. May, B.D. Horne, T.L. Bair, N.L. Hall, J.F. Carlquist, D.L. Lappe, and J.B. Muhlestein. "Relation of vitamin D deficiency to cardiovascular risk factors, disease status, and incident events in a general healthcare population." *American Journal of Cardiology*. Oct. 2010; 106(7): 963–8

Barbosa, V.M., E.A. Miles, C. Calhau, E. Lafuente, P.C. Calder. "Effects of fish oil containing lipid emulsion on plasma phospholipids fatty acids, inflammatory markers, and clinical outcomes in septic patients: a randomized, controlled clinical trial." *Critical Care*, 2010; 14: R5.

Bolland, M.J., A. Avenell, J.A. Baron, A. Grey, G.A. MacLennan, G.D. Gamble, and I.R. Reid. "Effect of calcium supplements on a risk of myocardial infarction and cardiovascular events: Meta-analysis." *British Medical Journal*, 2010; 341: c3691.

Don, Y., S. Stallmann-Jorgensen, N.K. Pollock, R.A. Harris, D. Keeton, Y. Huang, K. Li, R. Bassali, D. Guo, J. Thomas, G.L. Pierce, J. White, M.F. Holick, and H. Zhu. "A 16-week randomized clinical trial of 2000 International Units daily vitamin D3 supplementation in Black youth: 25-hydroxyvitamin D, adiposity, and arterial stiffness." *Journal of Clinical Endocrinology & Metabolism*, 2010; 95(10): 4584–4591.

Lavie, C.J., J. H. Lee, and R. V. Milani. "Vitamin D and Cardiovascular Disease: Will It Live Up to its Hype?" *Journal of the American College of Cardiology*, 2011; 58; 1547–1556.

Leon, H., M.C. Shibata, S. Sivakumaran, M. Dorgan, T. Chatterley, R.T. Tsuyuki. "Effect of fish oil on arrhythmias and mortality: Systematic review." *The British Medical Journal*, 2008; 337: a2931.

Makhija, N., C. Sendasgupta, U. Kiran, R. Lakshmy, M.P. Hote, S.K. Chourhary, B. Airan, and R. Abraham. "The role of oral coenzyme Q10 in patients undergoing coronary artery bypass graft surgery." *Cardiothoracic and Vascular Anesthesia*, Dec. 2008; 22(6): 832–839.

Schaars. C.F. and A.F. Stalenhoef. "Effects ubiquinone (coenzyme Q10) on myopathy in statin users." *Current Opinion in Lipidology*, Dec. 2008; 19(6): 553–557.

Shargorodsky, M., O. Debby, Z. Matas, and R. Zimlichman. "Effect of long-term treatment with antioxidants (vitamin C, vitamin E, coenzyme Q10 and selenium) on arterial compliance, humoral factors and inflammatory markers in patients with multiple cardiovascular risk factors." *Nutrition & Metabolism*, 2010; 7: 55.

About the Author

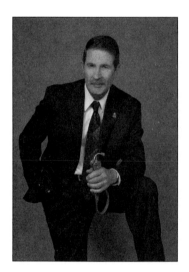

Michael Ozner, MD, FACC, FAHA, is one of America's leading advocates for heart disease prevention. Dr. Ozner is a board-certified cardiologist, a Fellow of both the American College of Cardiology and the American Heart Association, Medical Director of Wellness and Prevention at Baptist Health South Florida, and a well-known regional and national speaker in the field of preventive cardiology. He is symposium director for "Cardiovascular Disease Prevention," an annual international meeting dedicated to the treatment and prevention of heart attack and stroke. He was the recipient of the 2008 American Heart Association Humanitarian Award and was elected one of the "Top Cardiologists in America" by the Consumer Council of America. Dr. Ozner is also the author of *The Miami Mediterranean Diet* and *The Great American Heart Hoax.*

To contact Dr. Ozner, visit www.drozner.com.

Index

The letter t following a page number denotes a table or sidebar.

Abdominal aortic aneurysms, 22t
Abdominal obesity, 93t, 122, 148
Acne, omega-3 deficiency and, 73t
Active Living Initiative (CDC), 32t
Addiction, alcohol, 79t
Adrenaline, as stress hormone, 37
Adventist Health Study, on nuts and heart health, 78t
Aerobic exercise, 26, 28
Air quality, heart health and, 123–125
Alcohol consumption:
  benefits, 77–79
  caveats, 78–79
  guidelines, 79t
  HDL-raising properties, 117
  as hypertension risk, 132
  and sleep apnea, 49t
  tips for, 79t
Allergies:
  and Mediterranean diet, 83t
  omega-3 deficiency and, 73t
Almond milk, 69
Almonds:
  Adventist Health Study, 78t
  benefits of, 69, 76
  as part of heart-healthy diet, 9
Alpha-linolenic acid, 74
Alzheimer's disease:
  grape juice and, 80
  Mediterranean diet and, 69, 83t, 85
  trans fats and, 60
American Association for Therapeutic Humor, 51
American College of Cardiology, on vitamin D deficiency, 16
American College of Sports Medicine (ACSM):
  "Exercise Is Medicine" program, 27t
  exercise recommendations, 28
American Diabetes Association, diagnostic criteria, 133
American Heart Association (AHA):
  on dental care, 17
  on depression, 41

"FIT Formula," 28
  on social isolation, 50
  on sodium intake, 131t
  on vitamin D, 143
American Journal of Cardiology, on NFL fitness study, 25–26
American Journal of Clinical Nutrition, on Mediterranean diet, 82
American Journal of Epidemiology, on pollution and heart health, 124
American Journal of Preventive Medicine, on walking for health, 30
American Medical Association (AMA), "Exercise Is Medicine" program, 27t
American Society of Nephrology, fructose study, 61
Angina pectoris, 146
Angiotension converting enzyme (ACE) inhibitors, 99, 132
Angiotension receptor blockers (ARBs), 132
Antibiotics, in cow's milk, 68
Antihypertensive agents, xi, 132
Antioxidants:
  biochemistry of, 127–129
  by color, 128t
  CoQ10, 145–146
  foods containing, 129t
  and olive oil, 73
Anxiety:
  exercise and, 27
  and Mediterranean diet, 83t
  and stress, 38
Apnea. *See* Sleep apnea, obstructive
ApoA1 protein, 15, 107
ApoB protein, 15, 106
Apple consumption, benefits of, 117
Archives of General Psychiatry:
  on anxiety health risk, 38
  on Mediterranean diet, 85
Archives of Internal Medicine:
  on Mediterranean diet studies, 84
  on napping and heart health, 46
Arrhythmias:
  magnesium and, 144
  potassium and, 144

thyroid disorders and, 14
and weight loss, 87
Arterial elasticity:
  age-related hypertension, 130–131
  exercise and, 22
  and grape juice, 80
  laughter and, 51
Arthritis:
  chronic inflammation, 123
  exercise and, 27t
  IL-6 biomarker, 45
  omega-3 deficiency and, 73t
Asanas, 45
Aspirin:
  anti-clotting properties, 124t, 149
  as anti-inflammatory, 124t, 149
  benefits of supplemental, 148–150
  caveats, 149t, 150
  post–heart attack, 100
Asthma:
  and Mediterranean diet, 83t
  omega-3 deficiency and, 73t
Athens Medical School, on laughter and artery
  health, 51
Atherosclerosis:
  biochemistry of, 106–110
  in children, 57
  defined, xi
  and monounsaturated fat, 73–74
  reversing, 110–111, 122t
  Western diet link, 65
Atorvastatin, 119
Autoimmune diseases:
  chronic inflammation, 123
  and Mediterranean diet, 83t

Bair, Tami L., 16
Beans, benefits of, 76
Beef, caveats, 62–68
Behavioral therapy:
  for diabetics, 136
  for panic attacks, 39
  for smoking cessation, 11
  for stress relief, 38
Benson, Herbert, 42
Beta-amyloid peptides, 80
Beta blockers, 100, 132
Blood chemistry:
  blood pressure, 130–132
  blood sugar, 132–137
  case study, 91–105
    lab results after intervention, 101t–105t
    lab results before intervention, 94t–98t
  cholesterol, 111–119
  free radicals, 125–129, 130t
  heart attack genesis, 106–110
  importance of testing, 89–91
  inflammation, 120–125
  omega-3 levels, 137
  optimal values, 137–138, 138t
  reversing high-risk, 110–111
  vitamin D levels, 137

Blood clotting:
  and aspirin therapy, 124t
  and cinnamon, 82
  exercise and, 23t
  and grape juice, 80
  inflammation and, 120
  and olive oil, 73
  and stress, 37
  trans fats and, 60
Blood pressure, 130–132. *See also* Hypertension
  controlling, 133t
  effect of pollution on, 125
  inflammation and, 120
  in metabolic syndrome, 93t
  normal versus high, 130t
Blood sugar levels, 132–137. *See also* Diabetes
Blood tests. *See also* Blood chemistry
  importance of, 89–91
  optimal profile, 138t
  specific recommended, 13–16
Body mass index (BMI):
  calculating, 56
  and NFL fitness study, 25–26
Bone health, 27t. *See also* Osteoporosis
Boston University School of Medicine, yoga and
  health study, 45
Brain, Behavior and Immunity, on depression-
  inflammation link, 41
Breast cancer:
  and alcohol consumption, 78–79
  Mediterranean diet and, 84
  and soy milk, 69
  and vitamin B9, 78–79
Breathing:
  sleep apnea, 48–49
  as stress antidote, 42, 43t, 45
British Medical Journal:
  on diabetes and diet, 136
  on weight control via exercise, 30
Bronchitis, chronic inflammation, 123

Caffeine, as hypertension risk, 132
Calcium channel blockers, 132
Campbell, T. Colin, 67
Cancer:
  alcohol and, 79t
  and dairy products, 68t
  exercise and, 20, 27
  and fresh produce, 74
  and meats, 63–64, 65–66, 68
  and Mediterranean diet, 69, 82, 83t, 84
  and obesity, 56, 57t
  omega-3 deficiency and, 73t
  trans fats and, 60
Canola oil, 74t
Cardiovascular blood tests, 13–16
Castelli, William, 111t
Centers for Disease Control (CDC):
  Active Living Initiative, 32t
  on childhood obesity, 57
  dental care survey, 18
Checkups, routine:

dental exams, 17
physical exams, 12–16
Chemistry panel, 13
Chest pain, 146
China Study, The (Campbell), 67t
Cholesterol. *See also* HDL; LDL
    and almonds, 76
    blood chemistry, 111–119
    blood tests for, 14, 15-16
    and cinnamon, 82
    and dairy products, 68
    effect of diet on, 67t, 116–118
    effect of exercise on, 23, 29, 118
    effect of laughter on, 51
    effect of statins on, xi, 119
    effect of stress on, 37
    and fats, 59, 60
    and grape juice, 80t
    and meats, 63, 64, 67t
    medications for, 118–119
    Mediterranean diet and, 84, 117–118
    in metabolic syndrome, 93t
    and obesity, 57t
    and olive oil, 73
    optimal, 1, 111, 115t, 117, 138t
    and red wine, 77–78
    and whey protein, 148
Cigarettes. *See* Smoking cessation
Cinnamon, benefits of, 82
Circulation (AHA journal):
    on depression and heart health, 41
    on meat consumption risk, 64
    on processed meats, 66
Coenzyme Q10 (CoQ10), 145–146
Cognitive function. *See* Memory
Columbia University Medical Center,
    Mediterranean diet studies, 85
Complete blood count (CBC), 13. *See also* Blood
    chemistry
Continuous positive airway pressure
    (CPAP), 49
Cooking oils, caveats, 59t, 61t
Cortisol, 37, 51
Counseling. *See* Behavioral therapy
CPAP, 49
Craven, Lawrence, 148
C-reactive protein (CRP):
    blood tests for, 14
    reducing via socialization, 50
    reducing via yoga, 45
Crestor, 110, 119

Dairy products, caveats, 65t, 68–69
Dental care:
    importance of, 17–18
    periodontal inflammation, 123
Depression:
    alcohol and, 79t
    exercise and, 27
    and Mediterranean diet, 83t, 85
    omega-3 deficiency and, 73t
    and stress, 39–41

Diabetes:
    and air pollution, 125
    alcohol consumption and, 78
    biochemistry of, 132–136
    blood tests for, 13
    cinnamon and, 82
    and dairy products, 68t
    and exercise, 20, 21, 26, 30
    as heart attack risk, 135–137
    IL-6 biomarker, 45
    increasing incidence of, xi
    and LDL particle numbers, 114, 116t
    meats and, 63t, 66
    and Mediterranean diet, 69, 83t
    and obesity, 56, 57t
    omega-3 deficiency and, 73t
    and periodontal disease, 18
    and sleep quality, 48–49, 49t
    and stress, 37
    as stroke risk, 24
    symptoms of, 135t
    trans fats and, 60
    types of, 134
    vinegar and, 74
    whole grains and, 75–76
Diabetes Care, on air pollution factors, 125
Diabetes Prevention Program (DPP), 135–136
Diastolic pressure, defined, 22, 130
Diet:
    cholesterol-lowering, 116–119
    diabetic, 135–136
    glycemic food index, 135, 136t
    and heart disease, 2–3, 7–9, 67t, 69, 82, 83–84
    and hypertension, 131–132
    Mediterranean-style, 7–9, 69–86
        alcohol, grape juice, 79–80
        benefits of, 69–72, 82–85
        cinnamon, 82
        fish, 76–77
        fruits/vegetables, 74–75
        nuts/beans, 76
        olive oil, 73–74
        omega-3 fats, 72–73
        tea, 81
        vinegar, 74
        versus Western, 7–10, 67t, 69
        whole grains, 75–76
    potassium-rich foods, 145t
    super foods, 9t
    toxic versus healthy, 2–3, 6, 67t
    weight issues, 56–58, 86–88
    Western-style
        dairy products, 68–69
        fats, 58–61
        health risks of, 2–3, 55, 58
        high-fructose corn syrup, 61–62
        inflammation and, 122–123
        meats, 62–68
        versus Mediterranean, 7–10, 67t, 69
        weight issues, 55, 58–69
Drory, Yaacov, 11
Drugs. *See* Medications

East-West Study, diabetes–heart disease link, 135
Electrolytes, testing for, 13
Endorphins:
    exercise and, 27
    and laughter, 52
    as stress reliever, 41
Endothelial function, 80, 146
Environmental toxins, risks from, 123–125
Equal, calorie-free sweetener, 72t
European Heart Journal:
    on benefits of fresh produce, 74
    on panic attacks, 39
European Journal of Clinical Nutrition, on vinegar–blood sugar link, 74
European Society of Cardiology, on ruminant trans fats, 65t
Exams, physical. *See* Checkups, physical
Exercise. *See also* Fitness
    benefits of, 20–22, 25, 27
    cholesterol-lowering, 118
    for depression, 41
    and diabetes, 136
    FIT formula, 29
    fitness plans, 32t–33t
    and heart attacks, 23–24
    for hypertension, 22–23
    isometric, 30
    physician clearance for, 12,
    and strokes, 24–25
    tips for, 29–33
    walking, 29–30

Fats, dietary, 58–61
Fiber, benefits of, 70–71
Fish oil:
    benefits of, 76–77
    caveats, 77
    supplemental, 147
Fitness. *See also* Exercise
    defined, 19–20
    routines for, 29–33
    sample plans, 32t–33t
Folic acid (vitamin B9), 78–79
Food. *See* Diet
Framingham Offspring Study, 114
Framingham Study, cholesterol–heart attack link, 111
Free radicals, 108–110, 125–129, 130t
Friendship. *See* Social isolation
Fructose. *See* High-fructose corn syrup
Fruits, fresh:
    benefits of, 74–75
    as part of heart-healthy diet, 9
    suggestions for, 75t, 128t

Gallbladder disease, 57t
Gamma-aminobutyric acid (GABA), 45
Gestational diabetes, 134
GI disturbances:
    aspirin-related, 149t
    milk-related, 68t
Gingivitis. *See* Dental care

Glucose:
    ADA guidelines, 133t
    biochemistry of, 132–133
    in metabolic syndrome, 93t
    testing for, 13
Glycemic food index, 135, 136t
Grape juice, benefits of, 79–80
Gratz University (Austria), laughter therapy, 52

Harvard School of Public Health:
    fish consumption, benefits of, 77t
    meat consumption, health risks, 64, 66
    napping study, 46
    rice-diabetes link study, 76
Harvard University:
    Mediterranean diet, 84
    stress management, 42
    stroke study, 24, 29
HDL. *See also* Cholesterol
    blood tests for, 14–16
    improving, 116–119
    non-HDL cholesterol, 111–112
    and olive oil, 73
    optimal, 1, 115t, 138t
Heart attacks:
    aspirin as preventive, 124t
    biomedical genesis of, 106–110
    case study, 91–105
    exercise and, 20, 23–24
    and hypertension, 22t, 132
    Mediterranean diet and, 9, 84
    and obesity, 56, 57t
    pollution and, 123–125
Heart disease:
    blood tests indicative of, 12–16
    case studies, 5–7, 91–105
    causes, xi–xii
        biochemical/metabolic, 89–91
        cholesterol, 111–119
        dental factors, 17–18
        diabetes, 135–137
        diet, 2–3, 7–9, 58, 67t
        free radicals, 125–129
        hypertension, 130–132
        inflammation, 120–125
        nutritional deficiencies, 141–148
        omega-3 deficiency, 73t, 137
        smoking, 10–11
        stress, 35–36
        vitamin D deficiency, 137, 142–143
    mortality rates, xi, 2, 6, 67t, 91t
    reversing, 110–111
    risk-reduction checklists
        week 1, preventive measures, 18t
        week 2, exercise, 33
        week 3, stress management, 53t
        week 4, diet, heart-healthy, 88t
        week 5, blood chemistry, improving, 139t
        week 6, supplements, nutritional, 151t
Hemoglobin, measuring, 13, 133
Hennekens, Charles, 24

Heterocyclic amines (HCAs), 65–66
    High-density lipoprotein. *See* HDL
High-fructose corn syrup, 61–62
High-sensitivity C-reactive protein (hs-CRP), 14,
    120–122
Hippocrates, 148
HMG-CoA reductase inhibitors, 119. *See also*
    Statins
Hollis, (**AU query: First name? Not in text or
    Bib.**), 80
Hot Reactors, defined, 37–38
Humor. *See* Laughter, as stress antidote
Hunter, Gary, 26
Hydrogenation, 59
Hyperlipidemia, familial, 114, 117
Hypertension:
    and alcohol consumption, 78
    causes and cures, 130–132
    CoQ10 and, 146
    diseases caused by, 22t
    exercise and, 22–23, 26
    fructose and, 61–62
    grape juice and, 80, 80t
    magnesium and, 144
    meat and, 63t, 64
    medications for, 132
    and meditation, 44
    and Mediterranean diet, 69, 83t
    and obesity, 57t
    omega-3 deficiency and, 73t
    potassium and, 144
    and sleep apnea, 49t
    sodium and, 131t
    and stress, 37
    and stroke risk, 22t, 24
Hypertension Optimal Treatment study, 149–150

Ibuprofen, caveats, 124t
Impaired fasting glucose (IFG), 48
Indiana University-Purdue University Indianapolis
    (IUPUI), depression-inflammation link, 41
Inflammation:
    biochemistry of, 120–125
    cinnamon and, 82
    and depression, 41
    grape juice and, 80t
    meat and, 63t
    olive oil and, 73
    omega-3 and, 62
    reducing via diet, 69, 122–123
    reducing via exercise, 25
    reducing via socialization, 50
    reducing via yoga, 45
    red wine and, 77–78
    testing for, 120–121
    trans fats and, 60
    tumor necrosis factor (TNF), 129
Inflammatory bowel disease:
    chronic inflammation, 123
    and Mediterranean diet, 83t
    omega-3 deficiency and, 73t
Insomnia, alcohol-related, 79t

Institute of Medicine:
    exercise prescription, 21
    vitamin D guidelines, 142–143
Insulin:
    effects of exercise on, 30
    function of, 133–135
    LDL particles and, 16, 114
    sleep quality and, 47–48
    vinegar and, 74
INTER-HEART study, on alcohol consumption, 78
Interleukin-6 (IL-6):
    and depression, 41
    reducing through yoga, 45
    reducing via socialization, 50
Intermountain Medical Center Heart Institute
    (Murray, Utah), 16
International Agency for Cancer Research, 10t,
Internet resources:
    Active Living Initiative, 32t
    smoking cessation, 11
Isolation, social. *See* Social isolation
Isometric exercise, defined, 30

Journal of Clinical Endocrinology & Metabolism, on
    effects of resveratrol, 128–129
Journal of the American College of Cardiology, on
    smoking risks, 11
Journal of the American Medical Association, on
    fish consumption and heart health, 77t
*Journal of the Federation of American Societies for
    Experimental Biology,* on effects of resveratrol,
    129

Karolinska Institute (Stockholm), on
    inflammation, 120
Katzmarzyk, Peter T., 30
Keyes, Ancel, 9
Kidney function:
    blood tests for, 13
    hypertension and, 22t, 132
    and potassium, 144
    and sodium, 131t
    weight loss and, 87
    and whey protein, 148

Lancet, on exercise benefits, 23
Laughter, as stress antidote, 50–52
LDL. *See also* Cholesterol
    biochemistry of, 106–107
    blood tests for, 14–16
    effect of statins on, xi
    improving, 116–119
    and olive oil, 73
    optimal, 1, 115t, 117, 138t
    particle numbers, 111–114
LDL-P, 15, 113, 115, 122t, 138t
Licorice, hypertension and, 132
Lifestyle. *See also* Diet; Exercise
    benefits of active, 20–27
    effect on diabetes, 134–135
    effect on heart disease, xi–xii, 153
    elements of healthy, 153

inflammation-reducing, 121–122
risks of sedentary, 20–21, 93t, 117
toxic versus healthy, 2–4, 6–7
Lipid profile:
blood tests, 14
exercise and, 23t
optimal, 115t, 115–116
Lipitor, 119
Lipoprotein particles, measuring, 15
Liver function:
alcohol and, 79t
fructose and, 61
testing for, 13
Long Island Jewish Medical Center, air pollution study, 124
Low-density lipoprotein. See LDL
LPa test, 16
Lp-PLA2, 14, 120–122
Lung function, exercise and, 27t
Lyon Diet Heart Study, 83

Macrophages, defined, 110
Madden, Kenneth, 21
Magnesium, 144–145
Mayo Clinic, xii
Meat:
caveats, 62–68
recommendations, 67t
Medical College of Wisconsin, meditation and hypertension, 44
Medications:
anti-inflammatory, 121, 124t
blood pressure, 132
cholesterol-lowering, 118–119
for panic attacks, 39
post–heart attack, 99–100
and sleep apnea, 49t
smoking-cessation, 11
for stress, 38
Meditation, 43–44
Mediterranean diet:
alcohol, 77–79
Alzheimer's risk reduction, 85
antioxidant-rich, 128t, 129t
benefits of, 69–72, 82–87
and cancer protection, 84
and cardiovascular health, 83–84
cinnamon, 82
depression risk reduction, 85
and diabetes, 136–137
fish, 76–77
food/lifestyle pyramid, 70t
fruits/vegetables, 74–75
grape juice, 79–80
nuts/beans, 76
olive oil, 73–74
omega-3 fats, 72–73
tea, 81
vinegar, 74
versus Western, 7–10, 69
whole grains, 75
Meet the Press, 1

Memory:
and alcohol, 79t
exercise and, 27t
and grape juice, 80
Mediterranean diet and, 85
and napping, 47
and sleep apnea, 49
Mercury, in fish, 77
Metabolic syndrome:
blood tests for, 13, 15-16
defined, 93t
exercise and, 30
increasing incidence of, xi
and LDL particle numbers, 114
and Mediterranean diet, 69, 83t
Metformin, 136
Miami Mediterranean Diet, The (Ozner), 71t, 86
Milk. See Dairy products, caveats
Miller, Michael, 51
Mind-Body Institute (Boston), 42
Morris, Jeremy, 21
Mt. Sinai School of Medicine, cognitive benefits of grape juice, 80
Multiple sclerosis, dairy products and, 68t
Myeloperoxidase, 14, 126

Napping, benefits of, 46–47
NASA study, effect of napping on pilot performance, 47
National Cancer Institute, risks of meat consumption, 63
National Cholesterol Education Program, 111, 117t
National Football League (NFL), fitness study, 25–26
National Health Interview Survey, sleep quality and heart health, 47
National Heart, Lung and Blood Institute, 41, 50
National Stroke Association, 24
Neurodegenerative diseases, Mediterranean diet and, 83t
New England Journal of Medicine:
on aspirin's health benefits, 149
on pollution-caused heart disease, 123
New York University, dental care survey, 18
Niacin, 119
NIH-AARP Diet and Health Study, 84
Nitrosamines, 64
Nitrous oxide, 80, 120
Non-HDL cholesterol, 111–112
NSAIDs, caveats, 124t
Nutrition. See Diet
Nuts, benefits of, 76

Oatmeal, as part of heart-healthy diet, 9
Obesity. See also Weight issues
abdominal, 93t, 122, 148
BMI, calculating, 56
chronic inflammation, 123
exercise and, 20, 25–26
health risks associated with, 57t
and LDL particle numbers, 113–114
in metabolic syndrome, 93t
and sleep apnea, 49t

weight-loss tips, 86–88
Western diet and, 58–61
Obesity (journal), on weight and exercise study, 26
Obstructive sleep apnea. *See* Sleep apnea, obstructive
Ohio State University, yoga-for-health study, 45
Olive oil:
  benefits of, 73–74
  as part of heart-healthy diet, 9
Omega-3 fat:
  benefits of, 71, 72–73
  in Canola oil, 74t
  deficiencies in, 73t, 137
  in fish oil, 76, 117, 147
  versus omega-6 fat, 63
Omega-3 index, 16
Oral health. *See* Dental care
Osteoarthritis, obesity and, 56, 57t
Osteoporosis, 27t, 31
Oxidation, defined, 109

Pancreas, role in diabetes, 133–134
Pancreatitis, triglycerides and, 115
Panic attacks, 39
Pennington Biomedical Research Center, walking study, 30
Periodontal disease. *See* Dental care
Physical exams, routine, 12–16
Physicians Health Study (US):
  on aspirin's health benefits, 149
  on fish oil and heart health, 77t, 147
Phytochemicals:
  benefits of, 142
  in fresh produce, 74
  in whole grains, 75
Phytoestrogens, in soy milk, 69
Plaque formation, atherosclerotic, 106–110
Pollution, chronic inflammation and, 123–125
Popkin, Barry M., 64
Potassium, 144, 145t
Power nap, defined, 47
Processed meats, 66
Prostatitis, chronic inflammation and, 123
Psychosomatic Medicine, on yoga for health, 45
Pure Via, 72t

Quebec Cardiovascular Study, 16

Red meat, caveats, 62–68
Red wine, 77–78, 128–129
Relaxation response, 42, 43t
Resistance training, 26, 30–31
Resveratrol, 78, 128–129
Rosuvastatin, 119
Rudel, Lawrence, 73
Runner's high, 27
Russert, Tim, 1, 108

Salicin, 148
Salmon:
  benefits of, 76–77
  as part of heart-healthy diet, 9

Salt, excessive, 131t, 132
Saturated fats, 58–59
Scarmeas, Nikolaos, 85
Seven Countries Study, 8–9
Shah, Neomi, 49
Simvastatin, 119
Singh Indo-Mediterranean Diet Study, 84
Sinha, Rashmi, 63
SLEEP (journal), on sleep quality and heart health, 47
Sleep apnea, obstructive:
  and obesity, 57t
  risk factors, 49t
Sleep quality:
  alcohol and, 79t
  exercise and, 27
  stress management, 47–50
Smoking:
  and sleep apnea, 49t
  as stroke risk factor, 24
Smoking cessation:
  effect on heart disease, xi, 10–11
  tips for, 11t
Social isolation, as stressor, 50
Sodium:
  excessive, 131t, 132
  potassium and, 143–144
Soy milk, 68–68
Spek, Viola, 40
Splenda, 72t
State University of New York, sleep-deprivation study, 48
Statins:
  cholesterol-lowering, 119
  CoQ10 and, 146
  effect on heart disease, xi
  fish oil and, 147
  post–heart attack, 99
  reversing atherosclerosis, 110–111
Stevia, 62, 72t
Strauss, Sheila, 18
Stress:
  anger and, 37–38
  anxiety and, 38
  depression and, 39–41
  exercise and, 23t
  as health risk factor, 35–37
  hormonal response to, 36–37
  Hot Reactor quiz, 38t
  managing, 42–53
    via laughter, 50–52
    via meditation, 43–44
    via napping, 46–47
    via relaxation response, 42, 43t
    via sleep quality, 47–50
    via social interaction, 50
    via yoga, 44–46
  panic attacks and, 39
Stroke: Journal of the American Heart Association, on stroke study, 29
Strokes:
  and alcohol consumption, 78

defined, 24
exercise and, 20, 24–25, 29
and hypertension, 22t, 132
IL-6 biomarker, 45
low-dose aspirin and, 149
and obesity, 56, 57t
Sugar:
avoiding, 71–72
substitutes, 72t
Supplements and vitamins:
benefits of, 141–142
coenzyme Q10, 145–146
fish oil, 147
low-dose aspirin, 148–150
magnesium, 144–145
potassium, 143–144, 145t
vitamin B9, 78–79
vitamin D, 16, 137, 142–143
whey protein, 147–148
Support groups, 12
Sutanoff, Steve, 51
Sweet'N Low, 72t
Systolic pressure, defined, 22, 130

Tea, benefits of, 81
Teeth care. See Dental care
Thermogenesis, 71, 148
Thrombosis. See Blood clotting
Thyroid function, testing for, 13
Tobacco, smokeless, 10t. See also Smoking
     cessation
Transcendental meditation, 44
Trans fats, 58–60
caveats, 59t, 65t
foods to avoid, 60t
Trichopoulos, Dimitrious, 46
Triglycerides:
exercise and, 23, 25
implications of elevated, 115
in metabolic syndrome, 93t
and obesity, 57t
testing for, 14
Truvia, 72t
TSH. See Thyroid function, testing for
Tumor necrosis factor (TNF), 129
Type D individuals, 40–41

Ubiquinone, 145
University College London, panic attack study, 39
University of Alabama, weight and exercise study, 26
University of British Columbia, arterial elasticity study, 21–22
University of Buffalo, resveratrol study, 128–129
University of Cincinnati College of Medicine, cognitive benefits of grape juice, 80
University of Maryland, effect of laughter on artery health, 51

University of North Carolina, and meat caveats, 64
University of Texas Southwestern Medical Center: fitness study, 25–26
meat-cancer link study, 66
University of Tilburg (Netherlands), depression and heart health, 40
University of Warwick / SUNY, sleep-deprivation study, 48
Unsaturated fats, 58–59

Vegetables, fresh:
benefits of, 74–75
suggestions for, 75t, 128t
Vinegar, benefits of, 74
Visceral fat, 26
Vita, Joseph, 80
Vitamin B9, 78–79
Vitamin D:
blood test for, 16
deficiencies in, 137
supplemental, 142–143

Wake Forest University, monounsaturated fat study, 73
Walking:
fitness programs, 29–30
tips for increasing, 30t
Web sites:
Active Living Initiative, 32t
smoking-cessation, 11
Weight issues. See also Obesity
body mass index (BMI), 56–57
and children, 57t, 57–58
exercise and, 25–26, 29–30
and grape juice, 80
losing pounds healthfully, 86–88
and Mediterranean diet, 69–72
and olive oil, 73
Western diet. See under Diet
West Virginia School of Medicine, sleep study, 47
Whey protein, 147–148
Whole grains:
benefits of, 75
suggestions for, 76t
Wine, red:
HDL-raising properties, 117
and heart health, 77–78
resveratrol in, 78, 128–129
Women's Health Study, aspirin's health benefits, 149

Yale University, sleep apnea study, 49
Yoga, 44–46

Zocor, 119